I0816216

The Abortion Companion

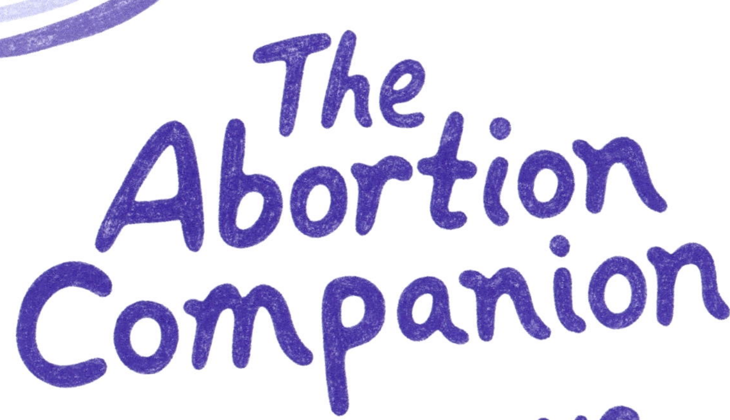

The Abortion Companion

an AFFIRMING HANDBOOK for YOUR CHOICE and YOUR JOURNEY

Becca Rea-Tucker
Illustrated by Jillian Barthold

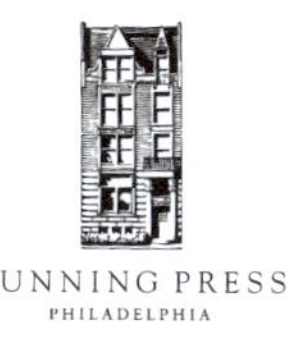

RUNNING PRESS
PHILADELPHIA

DISCLAIMER: This book is intended for adult readers. It is based solely on the opinions and ideas of the author on the subject matter of the book. The information contained in this book is intended for use as general information only and not for use in pursuing or recommending any treatment or course of action. It does not constitute medical or legal advice. The reader should consult a health or medical provider in all matters relating to their health. Certain sections of this book describe activities that could violate federal, state, or local laws and nothing in this book is intended to recommend any action that would cause anyone to do so. The author and publisher specifically disclaim all responsibility for any injury, loss, risk (personal or otherwise), legal consequence or incidental or consequential damage allegedly arising from any information or suggestions in this book.

Running Press
Hachette Book Group
1290 Avenue of the Americas, New York, NY 10104
www.runningpress.com
@Running_Press

First Edition: January 2026

Published by Running Press, an imprint of Hachette Book Group, Inc.
The Running Press name and logo are trademarks of Hachette Book Group, Inc.

The Hachette Speakers Bureau provides a wide range of authors for speaking events. To find out more, go to www.hachettespeakersbureau.com or email HachetteSpeakers@hbgusa.com.

Running Press books may be purchased in bulk for business, educational, or promotional use. For more information, please contact your local bookseller or the Hachette Book Group Special Markets Department at Special.Markets@hbgusa.com.

The publisher is not responsible for websites (or their content) that are not owned by the publisher.

Print book cover and interior design by Justine Kelley and Frances J. Soo Ping Chow

Library of Congress Control Number: 2024050466

ISBNs: 979-8-89414-101-5 (hardcover), 979-8-89414-102-2 (ebook)

Printed in China

TLF

10 9 8 7 6 5 4 3 2 1

Contents

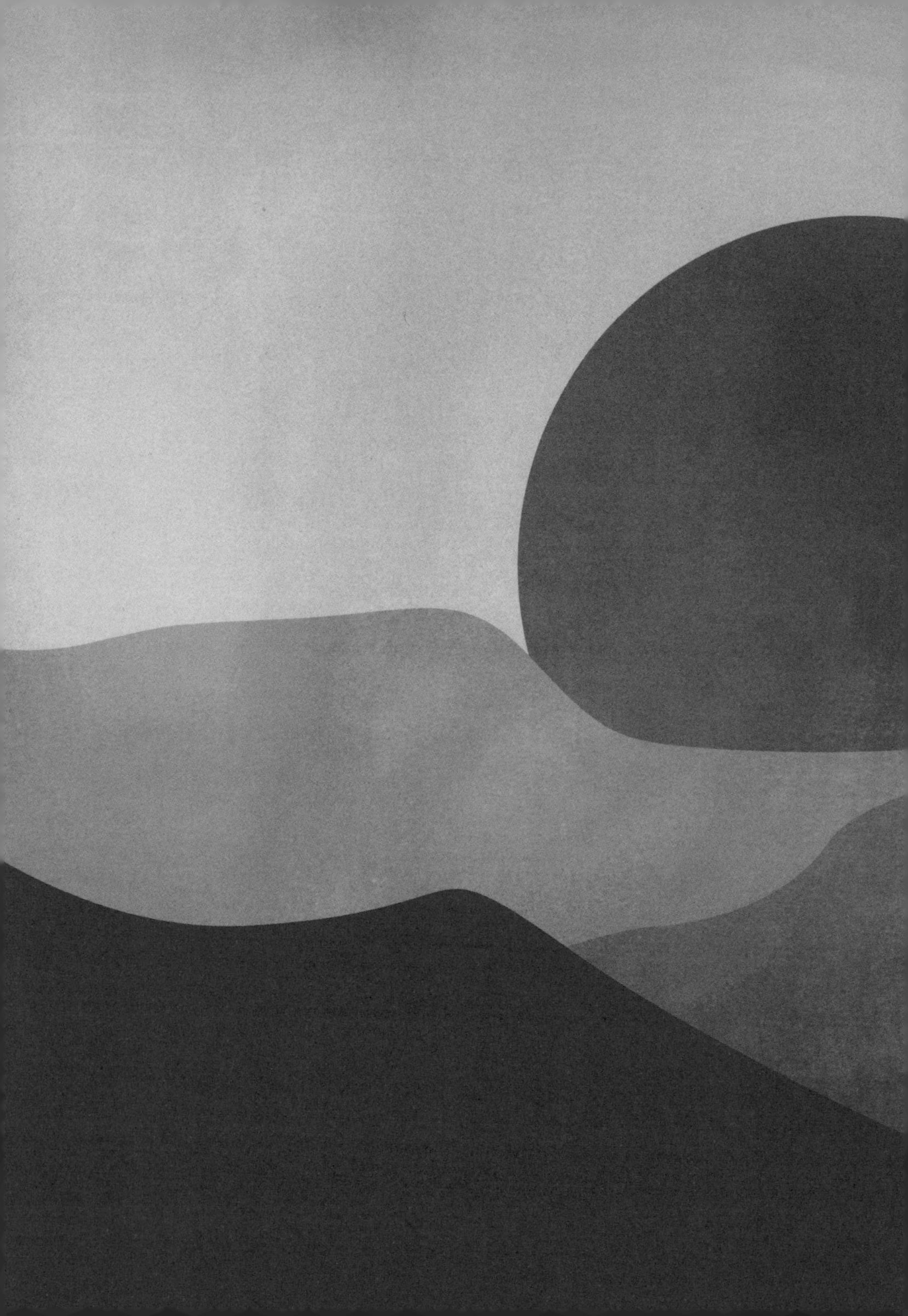

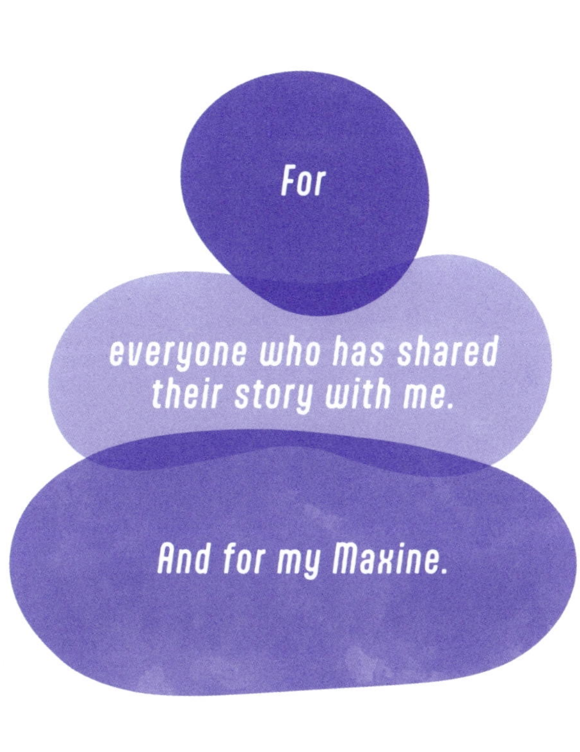
For
everyone who has shared
their story with me.
And for my Maxine.

WELCOME

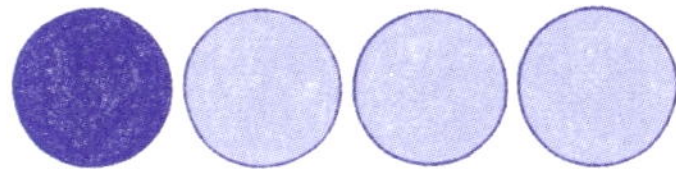

In case you've never heard anyone talk about their abortions before: Hi! I'm Becca, and I'm so glad you're here. I'm one of the one in four women* in the United States who have had or will have an abortion in their lifetime. Yes—one in four! I know this statistic might be surprising, but that's because anti-abortion stigma tries so hard to make us believe we're alone in our experiences.

I found out I was pregnant for the first time when I was in college. (Psst: You can read my abortion story on page 112.) I knew right away that I didn't want to continue the pregnancy. With the support of my then-boyfriend and an independent clinic, I had an abortion.

*Note: Trans men and nonbinary people have abortions too.

The morning after taking the abortion pills, I finally felt like I could breathe again. It was the most intense feeling of relief I could conjure.

I was certain that having an abortion was the right choice for me, and I never wavered on it. I was and am proud of how I cared for myself; I prioritized my life, my dreams. Still, the anti-abortion stigma was so powerful and so pervasive that I told almost no one about my abortion for years. I lived in fear of someone finding out. What if they judged me? What if they told everyone else?

Over time, I connected with other people who have had abortions (mostly online at first!) and realized that I was very much not alone. I was so inspired by the compassion reproductive rights activists extend to others who have abortions and to themselves. I was energized by their unapologetic support, and eventually I decided to start sharing my own abortion story publicly. It took me a while, but I made it.

Having abortions is very common, but, unfortunately, so is experiencing shame about it. If you've had an abortion or you're contemplating one, and you've been lugging around the shame equivalent of some kind of large hiking backpack filled with rocks, I understand. The hardest part isn't always the abortion itself—it might be being pregnant when you don't want to be, hearing someone you love speak negatively about people who have abortions, or the isolation that comes from not feeling like you can talk about your experience.

This book is here to remind you that it's absolutely okay to have abortions, and that you are not alone. I hope it meets you wherever you are in your journey—whether you had an abortion ten days ago or ten years ago, whether you have an appointment scheduled soon or are simply considering your options. I wrote it to create a comfortable and affirming place for you to sort through your feelings and heal from the wounds inflicted by stigma. I like to think of it as an antidote to shame.

Everyone deserves unconditional compassion and support throughout their abortion experiences. But many of us are met with judgment instead. And even when we do receive support, it's often conditional—only given if we act appropriately remorseful or if our experience fits in with one of the few, narrow circumstances some people deem "acceptable" for having an abortion. But you don't have to regret or justify your abortion to want or benefit from support. I hope this book helps you feel confident in *all* your reproductive choices.

It's important to note: I don't worry about convincing anti-abortion people of anything. Many of them will continue to be anti-abortion regardless, and they are not the important ones in this conversation. This book is written specifically for us, people who have abortions. We deserve so much better, and we can have it.

There's a lot of bad information about abortion out there. Like *a lot.* It can be hard to find genuine support. If you google "abortion support," a lot of anti-abortion trash disguised as help pops up. You'll find results with neutral to positive sounding names like "Her Choice to Heal" or "Abortion Recovery Guide Workbook." Sounds good, right? They're not. On closer examination, many of these "resources" prey on people's need for support while offering half-truths and further shaming. This shit is insidious and intentional.

And even when it's not overtly anti-abortion, there's a lot of half-hearted, conditional support out there. Take for example the slogan "abortion should be safe, legal, and rare." It's not rare, has never been rare, and doesn't have to be rare. This kind of support translates into something like *Okay, yes, we'll support you—as long as you act appropriately remorseful. We'll support you—as long as you're not using abortion as birth control.* (This isn't a thing.) *We'll support you—as long as you regret it.* There's an overwhelming message that abortion should be an absolute last resort, and there's only one (appropriate) way to feel about it: ashamed. But you don't owe anyone shame in exchange for support.

There absolutely are good resources out there (check out the list on page 151!). But it's hard to find them when they're buried under so many bad ones.

This book is here to help you process your abortion experiences on your own terms, outside of the stigmatizing scripts we've been given. And I want you to know: This isn't a sad book! Sadness can be part of our abortion experiences, but the experience is usually a lot more nuanced. There's no particular way you *should* feel about your abortions, and here you'll find acceptance for all of your feelings—complicated or not.

Think of this book as your very own pro-abortion hypewoman to replace the negative voices that might be floating around in your head. It's a resource you can turn to whenever you need it, whether you're looking for information, comfort, or simply a reminder that you're not alone. And you don't have to read it in order! But if you *are* reading in order, we'll start by exploring the history of abortion in the United States, the current legal landscape, and the barriers, bans, and restrictions that make access more difficult by design.

This book uses guided exercises, self-reflective prompts, meditations, and affirmations to validate and support the full spectrum of abortion experiences. You'll also find tools to help you speak with your family and friends, ask for support, and actually accept it when it's offered.

My dream is for you to pass this book around. When someone tells you they need an abortion or need help with processing one, you'll have a recommendation ready. I hope that it helps you feel at peace with your path and confident in your decisions. I hope that you'll feel comfortable talking about abortion, without all the unnecessary shame.

There's nothing wrong with having abortions, and I'm so proud of you.

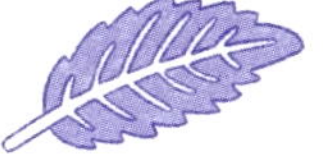

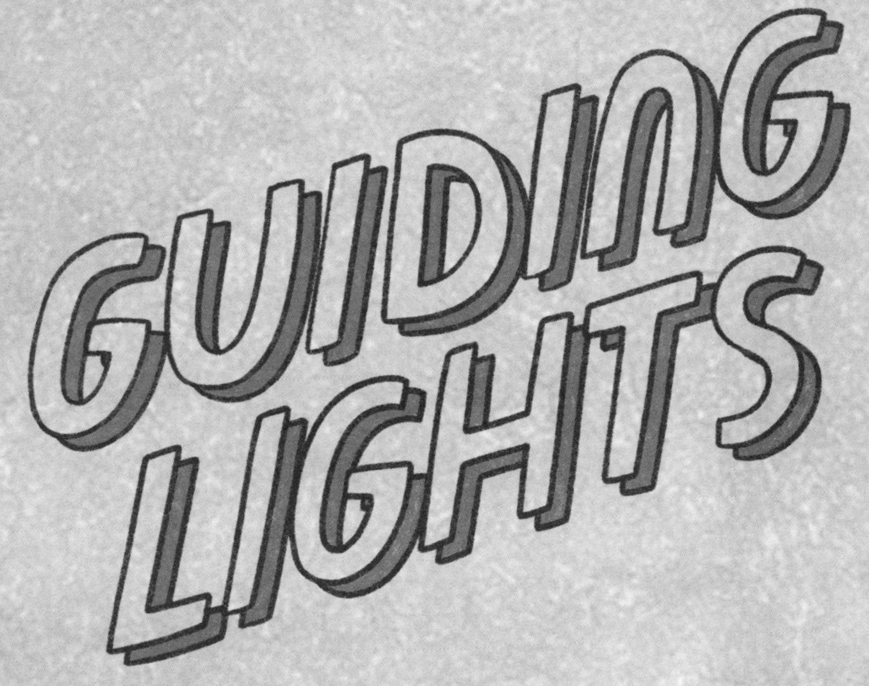
GUIDING
LIGHTS

Core beliefs that shape how I talk about abortion and the people who have them.

Abortion is common and normal.

People who have abortions deserve support, not shame or stigma.

There is no particular "kind of person" who has abortions—all kinds of people have them, in all kinds of circumstances.

There's no one-size-fits-all way to have an abortion, and there's no one-size-fits-all way to feel about your abortion. Any feelings you have about your abortion are 100 percent okay, even if they are complicated, even if they are conflicting.

Any reason for having an abortion
is the right reason.

Our right to safe abortion care in our communities
is inherent and non-negotiable.

I use non-gendered language because
people of all genders have abortions.

I use the term "pro-abortion" instead of "pro-choice." By saying abortion when we mean abortion, it helps to normalize people's experiences and decrease shame due to stigma. "Pro-choice" isn't meaningful if there isn't actually a choice due to restrictions, bans, and barriers, or if all choices aren't equally respected.

We have always had and will always have abortions.

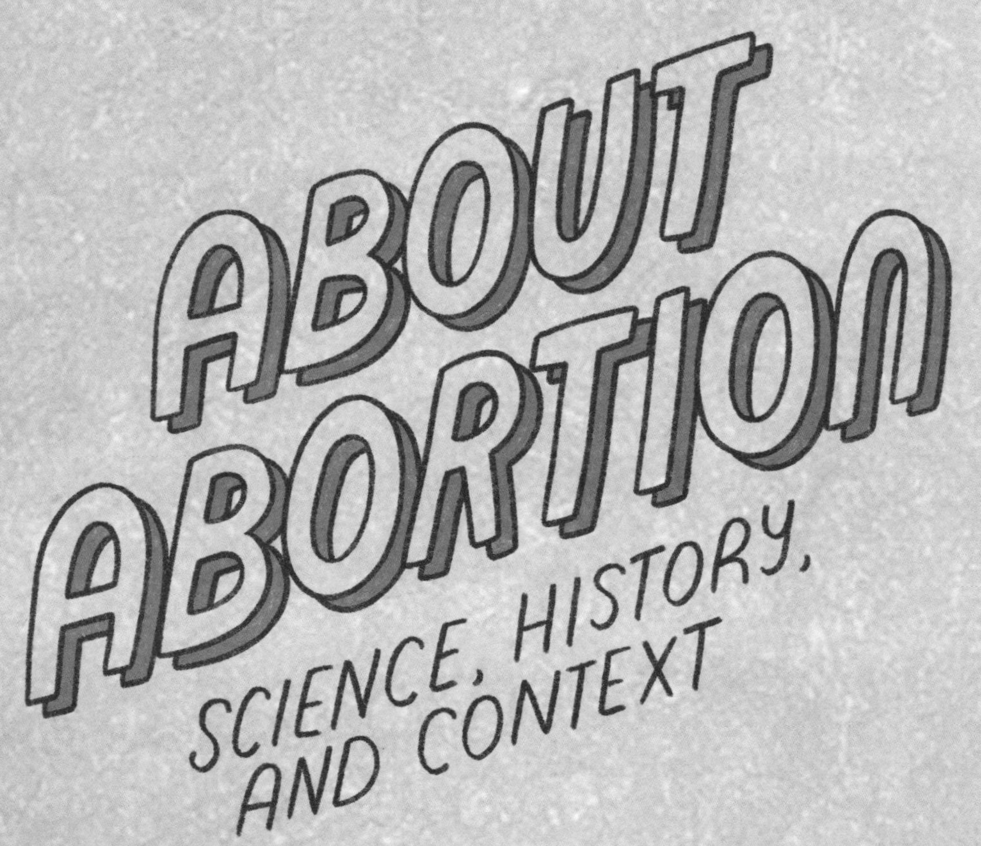
ABOUT ABORTION
SCIENCE, HISTORY, AND CONTEXT

Abortion 101

There's so much misinformation out there about abortion! Let's take a minute to go through the details so we're all on the same page.

So what *is* an abortion? Like, literally.*

An abortion is the termination of a pregnancy. A **spontaneous abortion** is when a pregnancy ends on its own, also called a miscarriage or early pregnancy loss. An **induced abortion** is when a person intentionally ends a pregnancy.† Spontaneous and induced abortions are treated medically in the same way.

A **medication abortion** is when medications (often abortion pills) are used to expel the pregnancy from the uterus. When we say "abortion pills," we're generally talking about the combination of mifepristone and misoprostol, but misoprostol can also be taken alone over multiple doses. Other forms of medication abortion include vaginal suppositories, muscular injections, and IV medications (including inductions at the hospital). Medication abortions make up the majority—almost

*Abortion 101 content has been reviewed by Dr. Ghazaleh Moayedi, abortion provider and board chair of Physicians for Reproductive Health.

†We don't use the terms "elective" or "therapeutic abortion" anymore because they're stigmatizing and not medically accurate.

two-thirds—of abortions in the United States. Abortion pills can be prescribed in person at a clinic or via telemedicine, and they can be used in a medical setting or at home. Pills can also be obtained outside of the medical system and used at home, which is called a **self-managed abortion (SMA)**.

A **procedural abortion** is when medical tools are used to remove the pregnancy from the uterus. Most procedural abortions happen in a clinic or hospital setting and use manual or electrical suction to remove the pregnancy. **Uterine aspiration** is a procedural abortion where suction alone is used. Uterine aspiration used to be called **dilation and curettage (D&C)**—and still might be called this—but curettage has not really been used as a method of procedural abortion for a couple of decades. **Dilation and evacuation (D&E)** procedures use a combination of suction and medical instruments to remove the pregnancy. This can be a two-day procedure because providers might use a medication like misoprostol or mifepristone, or insert osmotic dilators that absorb moisture to help stretch the cervical opening.

Pregnancies end in abortion for people who do not want to be pregnant, and they also end in abortion for people who want to remain pregnant but can't.

Most abortions happen during the first trimester. But some happen during the second or third trimester, called a **later abortion** (*not* a late-term abortion—we've also done away with this stigmatizing phrase!). Later abortions happen in all kinds of circumstances, but some common ones include the pregnant person not being able to access care where they live and needing to travel, needing time to come up with the money to afford care, finding out that the pregnancy is not progressing in a healthy way, not being able to take time off work or find childcare right away, not realizing they're pregnant until later in pregnancy, and having trouble accessing a judicial bypass (see page 24) if they're younger than eighteen.

Is it safe?

With a major complication rate of less than 1 percent, abortion is very medically safe. You might have been told otherwise, but having abortions does not increase your risk for breast cancer, infertility, depression, anxiety, or PTSD. Both mifepristone and misoprostol are safer than Tylenol. Additionally, experiencing a miscarriage and having an abortion by ingesting pills look clinically identical. If you're undergoing a medication abortion and you need to go to a doctor, you can simply say you are having a miscarriage—they will not be able to tell you took abortion pills (if they are not placed in the vagina).

While abortion is very medically safe, anti-abortion restrictions and bans continue to spread, so it can be *legally* risky. Depending on where you live, there might be state laws designed to make getting an abortion harder. These strategies include mandating ultrasounds, imposing waiting periods, forcing health providers to tell you biased and inaccurate information, and banning abortion after an arbitrary week of pregnancy. Because they compromise care, abortion restrictions and bans hurt all people who are pregnant—including those who have miscarriages or complications such as ectopic pregnancies. You can read more about barriers and how to navigate them on page 20.

What can I expect?

MEDICATION ABORTION

For most medication abortions, you will take a mifepristone pill first and then four to eight misoprostol pills twenty-four to forty-eight hours later. For most people this is a four- to six-hour process from taking the pills to passing the pregnancy. After taking the misoprostol pills, you might experience fever, chills, nausea, or diarrhea. You can expect slight, moderate, or intense cramping that can last for a while, and mild-heavy bleeding that may last for several days (and up to eight weeks). Many people feel most comfortable in the bathroom during this process.

PROCEDURAL ABORTION

Procedural abortions in the first trimester usually take five to fifteen minutes. You will lie down on a medical table with your legs in footrests. When you're ready, your provider will insert a speculum into your vagina (you can also ask to insert it yourself!) so they can see the cervix. They

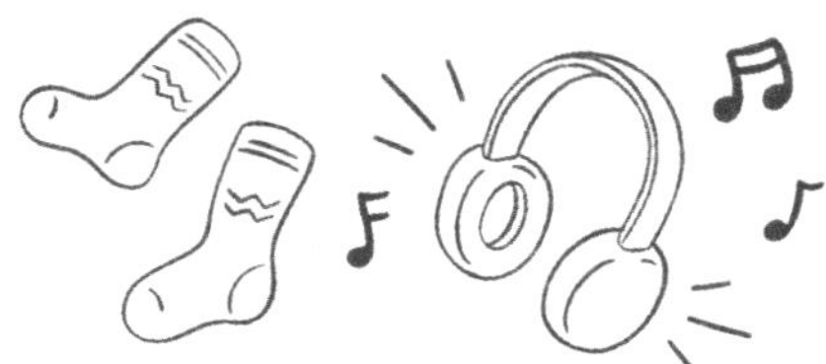

Some general tips for a procedural abortion:

- Wear comfortable clothes—a soft waistband, cozy socks, your comfort hoodie.
- Bring headphones, a snack, and a phone charger. Depending on the clinic's capacity to allow others in the room, you can have someone hold your hand throughout the procedure—this could be a loved one, a clinic staff member, or an abortion doula.
- If you have sedation, you will need someone to drive you home. You can listen to music or a podcast during the procedure or use earplugs.

Abortions later in pregnancy take more time, and the recovery might be different.

will apply a local anesthetic to the cervix to help reduce pressure and pain. Then they will use dilators to stretch open the cervix. They'll pass a small, sterile tube through the cervix into the uterus and use gentle suction to remove the pregnancy. They will use either manual suction or a suction machine, which makes a loud humming noise. You will probably be monitored in the clinic for a short time afterward. You can expect slight cramping and some spotting or bleeding.

Clinics offer different ways to help you stay comfortable during the procedure, including oral or IV medications, IV sedation, deep sedation, and general anesthesia. Ibuprofen, naproxen, and heating pads are good options for pain relief afterward (but not aspirin, which is a blood thinner!). It's a good idea to have supplies like pads (overnight or heavy flow) on hand. Feel free to send someone to get them for you!

Am I alone?

No matter what you've been told, abortion is very common, and all kinds of people have them. Currently, 15 to 20 percent of all pregnancies in the United States end in abortion. For unintended pregnancies (which make up about half of all pregnancies), the rate is even higher: 35 to 40 percent.

One in four women in the United States has had or will have an abortion in her lifetime—and this number doesn't reflect all abortions, because trans men and nonbinary people have abortions too. A 2023 study found that as many as 16 percent of people who have abortions identify as queer or trans, with 1 percent identifying as nonbinary or trans masc.

The majority of people who have abortions are already parenting. It is common to have multiple abortions—almost half of people having an abortion have had one before. More than half of people who have abortions in the United States identify as Christian.

People have abortions at all stages of pregnancy, for all kinds of reasons. Every single one of them is valid.

Reproductive Justice, Defined

Reproductive justice is a human rights framework that says that we deserve full and unquestioned autonomy over our bodies, and that we have the right to parent—or not—with support and safety, regardless of the political landscape, regardless of what any court decides. Originated by a group of visionary Black women at a conference in the early 1990s, the reproductive justice movement connects the ways race, class, and gender impact someone's ability to achieve reproductive liberation.

Abortion care falls under the reproductive justice umbrella.

Dr. Toni M. Bond Leonard

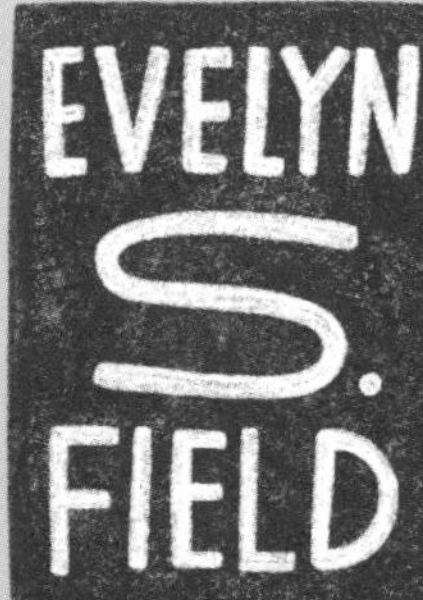

BISOLA MARIGNAY

CASSANDRA McConnell

Terri James

ELIZABETH TERRY

KIM YOUNGBLOOD

REVEREND ALMA CRAWFORD

"ABLE" MABLE THOMAS

WINNETTE P. WILLIS

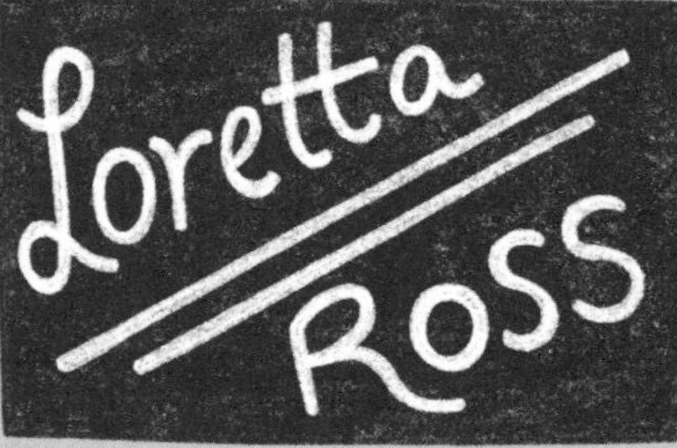

CYNTHIA NEWBILLE

I had an abortion in October of last year while I was on tour. I went to Planned Parenthood, where they gave me the abortion pill. It was easy. Everyone deserves that kind of access.

—*Phoebe Bridgers*

A Brief History of Abortion in the United States

Before 1803

No legal restrictions in the United States before "quickening"—the point at which the pregnant person reports movement.

1803

Britain's Lord Ellenborough's Act criminalized abortion even before quickening. Later, laws in the United States would copy the restriction.

1821

Connecticut became the first state to make having an abortion a criminal offense.

1830

New York made having an abortion chargeable as second-degree murder, with one exception: if the abortion was deemed medically necessary by two physicians.

1847

The American Medical Association (AMA) was formed.

1857

Dr. Horatio Storer (the *worst*) led a committee that argued that abortion in all instances was a criminal act.

1873

The Comstock Act made it illegal to send information about contraception or abortion through the mail.

1880

All states had laws in place to restrict abortion in some way.

1800s–1900s (throughout)

Midwives were pushed out and MDs were put in charge of prenatal care and childbirth.

Police conducted surveillance and raids on abortion providers.

Abortion care was provided illegally.

1910

All states had laws making abortion illegal at every stage in pregnancy, with some medical exceptions.

1964

The Association for the Study of Abortion was formed. Their work contributed to the success of the movement for decriminalization by framing abortion as a public health issue.

1967

As governor, Ronald Reagan legalized abortion in California, but only under certain medical circumstances.

1970

Hawaii became the first state to legalize abortion without a stated medical reason.

1973

The Supreme Court's ruling in *Roe v. Wade* legalized abortion nationwide but still allowed states to restrict abortion care based on potential viability, which is medically recognized as around 24 to 26 weeks.

1976

Congress passed the racist Hyde Amendment, which keeps federal dollars from being used to pay for abortion care, disproportionately impacting poor Black and Brown people enrolled in Medicaid. It made it much more difficult, if not impossible, to access care for those who could not afford to pay out of pocket.

1980

In *Harris v. McRae*, the Supreme Court ruled that states participating in Medicaid didn't have to pay for abortions.

1981

In *Bellotti v. Baird*, the Supreme Court ruled that pregnant minors can petition the court to have an abortion without notifying their parents.

1984

President Ronald Reagan introduced the Global Gag Rule, which prevents health organizations anywhere in the world that receive U.S. aid from providing abortion care, referrals, or information.

1988

Misoprostol, one of the two components of a medication abortion, was granted FDA approval.

1992

In *Planned Parenthood v. Casey*, the Supreme Court ruled that states could restrict abortion as long as there wasn't an "undue burden" placed on the pregnant person.

1994

The Freedom of Access to Clinic Entrances Act made it a federal crime to obstruct access to abortion clinics.

2000

Mifepristone, the other component of a medication abortion, was granted FDA approval.

2016

In *Whole Woman's Health v. Hellerstedt*, the Supreme Court struck down two restrictions on abortion care in Texas.

2021

The Texas law SB8 banned abortions in that state after six weeks of pregnancy and placed a $10,000 bounty on anyone who "aids and abets" abortion.

2022

In May, Justice Samuel Alito's draft opinion revealing that *Roe* would be struck down was leaked.

In June, the Supreme Court officially ruled on *Dobbs v. Jackson Women's Health Organization*, the case in which the court struck down the constitutional right to abortion.

Today and Forever

We (people who have abortions and our allies!) will work to make sure every pregnant person has access to the abortion care they deserve.

Barriers
(and Paths Around Them)

There are a lot of barriers to getting the care we need, by design. But there are also a lot of people and organizations ready to help. Let's break 'em down together.

Legal Barriers

Because abortion is often used as a political bargaining chip, there are constant legal attacks on access. *Roe v. Wade*, which protected abortion access in the United States at a federal level, was struck down in 2022, three-ish years before this book was published. At the time of publication, twelve states have total abortion bans in place, and twenty-nine more have restrictions to care. Psst: *That's forty-one states*. These restrictions take many forms.

There are the dusty, tried-and-true strategies used by anti-abortion lawmakers for decades:

The Hyde Amendment prevents federal Medicaid funding from being used to pay for abortions.

Fetal personhood laws strip away the bodily autonomy of pregnant people.

TRAP (targeted restrictions on abortion providers) laws impose unnecessary restrictions on abortion providers (like requiring hospital admitting privileges—an agreement that allows a provider to admit patients to the hospital and treat them there).

//////////////////////

Unnecessary burdens are placed on patients, like requiring they undergo mandatory ultrasounds, endure waiting periods, and/or be forced to listen to nonscientific misinformation provided by the state.

//////////////////////

Parental involvement laws limit young people's ability to make their own abortion decisions.

//////////////////////

Restrictions on healthcare for incarcerated people make accessing care very challenging or impossible.

//////////////////////

(How many times can I say "unnecessary" before it stops sounding like a word?)

And then there are new strategies popping up, like the worst possible game of Whac-A-Mole:

Placing a $10,000 bounty on anyone who allegedly "aids and abets" abortion (that is, helps someone access the care they need).

Prosecuting people for crossing state lines to have abortions or to help people have abortions.

Passing ordinances that forbid people from using certain city or county highways to drive someone to receive abortion care.

Note: All these examples are from my (current) home state of Texas.

How to Navigate Legal Barriers

We can have medically safe abortions regardless of legality, and no one should ever be criminalized for their pregnancy outcome. But people are—particularly Black and Brown people, poor people, disabled people, immigrants, and people in rural areas.

The majority of people who are criminalized for having abortions are reported to police by a healthcare worker or by someone they know. Don't use social media, email, or text messages to share info about your pregnancy or abortion with anyone—use an encrypted messaging app like Signal. Learn more about digital safety on page 39.

In the United States, you can call the Repro Legal Helpline at 844-868-2812 for information about legal risk and ways to protect yourself.

If you're under eighteen, some states* require that your parents be notified or give their consent before you can have an abortion; these are called parental involvement laws. If it's best for you not to have your parents

*As of publication time: Alabama, Arizona, Arkansas, Florida, Idaho, Indiana, Kansas, Kentucky, Louisiana, Massachusetts, Michigan, Mississippi, Missouri, Nebraska, North Carolina, North Dakota, Ohio, Oklahoma, Pennsylvania, Rhode Island, South Carolina, Tennessee, Texas, Utah, Virginia, Wisconsin, Wyoming

involved in your decision, you will need a judicial bypass. This is an order from a judge that allows a young person to have an abortion without the notification or consent of their parents. There are organizations that can help you figure this process out, and the Repro Legal Helpline (mentioned above) can help connect you.

Remember: Despite the constantly shifting legal landscape, abortion is here to stay.

Practical Barriers

Having an abortion can be expensive (especially if it happens later in pregnancy). You need enough money to pay for the care itself, but first you need enough money to get there.

As more states ban abortion and more clinics close, many of us are forced to travel farther from home to find care. And this means that costs rise: gas, flights, food, somewhere to stay, childcare, and lost wages from missed work. Abortion access should not depend on geography, but it often does.

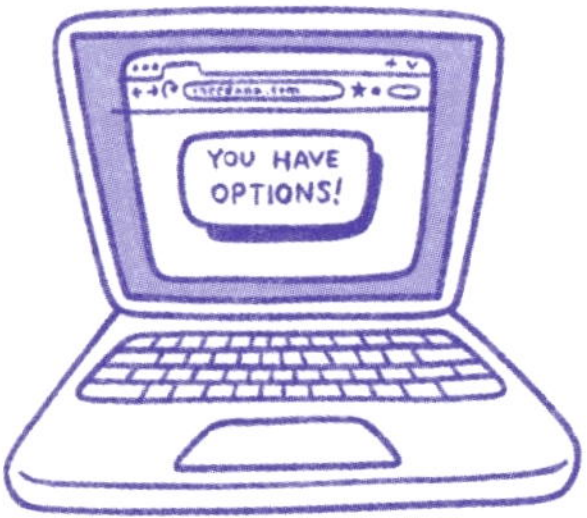

How to Navigate Practical Barriers

Visit I Need an A (www.ineedana.com) for up-to-date information about how to access abortion care at any stage of pregnancy. Unfortunately, Google (and its growing bevy of AI search tools) is not a reliable source for accurate information about abortion care. Anti-abortion organizations use search engine optimization strategies to rank highly in search results and targeted ads in order to boost misinformation. The result is that fake clinics are shown alongside real clinics, and accurate info about abortion is pushed further down.

Reach out to your local abortion fund or practical support organization! They can help pay for procedures, pills, travel, a place to stay, food, and childcare. They can also provide support with figuring out all the logistics.

Lean on your network—it's absolutely okay to ask for help! You can order abortion pills before you need them and keep them in your cabinet for up to two years.

Societal Barriers

Abortion stigma is everywhere—it shows up on TV and on billboards, from politicians, in the media, and even from people we love. It isolates us and tricks us into thinking that we're all alone. Even though we all love someone who's had an abortion, you might not know about it. And stigma creates a culture of fear that makes people feel uncomfortable asking for or offering help. That sucks!

How to Navigate Societal Barriers

It can be incredibly validating to find community with other people who have had abortions, online or in real life. Connecting with others reminds us that we're not alone and adds a super necessary layer of insulation against anti-abortion trash. Having abortions can feel incredibly isolating, but it doesn't have to.

I've mentioned elsewhere that before I had my abortion, I'd only ever heard one person's abortion story firsthand. Now, I'm honored to have heard hundreds (maybe thousands!). It can be incredibly healing to see your experiences reflected in someone else's. And I've found that listening to other people's abortion stories helps to break down and replace any shame-filled messaging that might be lingering in some forgotten corner of your brain.

The Fake Clinic Scam

Fake clinics (aka crisis pregnancy centers) are designed to try to stop people from having abortions through tricks and lies. They mimic real health centers, but they don't actually offer any health services. There are a lot of them (somewhere around 3,000 in the United States. And many of these garbage places are funded by taxpayer dollars that *should* go to the real clinics!

Some things they do:

Pressure you to have an ultrasound.
Note: You do not have to have one in order to have an abortion, except where required by state law if you're having your abortion via a clinic.

Lie to you about gestational age.

Lie to you about medical issues that allegedly happen after having abortions (for example, breast cancer, fertility issues, depression—none of these are scientifically linked to having abortions).

Lie to you about your options.

Tell you stories designed to scare and intimidate you.

Shame you about your sex life or sexuality.

Share your personal "intake" information with other anti-abortion organizations or even the police. They can do this because they're not licensed medical facilities and do not follow HIPAA regulations.

Waste your time and try to run out the clock until it's harder for you to access care.

Heads up: A fake clinic might have a similar name to a real clinic, be next door to one, or take over the building of one after it closes, so make sure you research carefully using an up-to-date source (more on that in the Resources section on page 151).

How to spot them/red flags:

Ads for free pregnancy tests or ultrasounds, but they don't mention any other real reproductive services (like birth control).

Billboards with unclear language about "help," "abortion alternatives," or "abortion reversal."

No information about actual abortion services on their website.

Affiliations with certain organizations such as Birthright International, Care Net, Heartbeat International, or National Institute of Family and Life Advocates.

How to make sure you aren't going to a fake clinic:

When you call clinics, ask directly and confirm that they actually provide abortion care.

//////////////////////

Ask your local abortion fund for recommendations.

//////////////////////

Visit www.ineedana.com for an up-to-date list of options based on where you live. Unfortunately, if you use Google, it will often show you fake clinics in the results.

//////////////////////

If you've spoken with or been to one of these places, I want to emphasize that you deserved so much better. You should have been presented with all your (real) options. You should never have been made to feel ashamed.

Stigma Lies

Getting rid of abortion stigma is in my top five goals in life.*

*The other goals mainly involve things like having a huge amount of fun with my baby, living in a house with a wraparound porch on a seaside cliff, and learning how to make my own paper.

Stigma is at the root of some really bad shit, and it tells us a lot of lies. It says that we really shouldn't have abortions, but if we do, then we have to at least be appropriately ashamed about it. It claims that having an abortion is a last resort that we only deserve in certain (and ever-changing) circumstances. None of that is true, but it can be pretty hard to believe because the stigma is *everywhere.*

We're constantly told abortion is generally immoral and unacceptable. And what else are we supposed to think when it's some form of illegal in forty-one states? Criminalization reinforces stigma and makes having abortions feel illicit when it isn't. And even if we're taught that it's *technically* okay, it's often in the sense that it's okay for *other people.* It's nearly impossible for me to imagine now, but a past version of me actually uttered the phrase, "Of course abortion is okay, but *I* could never have one." Like, ma'am, *why not*? There's a really long answer to that, but here's the short version. Society insists that there are two categories: the kind of people who have abortions and the kind of people who don't. This distinction is a total myth.

In my dream world, abortion would be presented as such a normal part of life that it seems to have always existed in our consciousnesses. But when I was growing up, I only heard abortion spoken about in hushed and allegedly appropriately reverent tones. Who wants to share their abortion story if there's a good chance it'll be met with judgment? Because it's rare for people to talk openly about their abortions, having abortions seems much rarer than it actually is. And when we don't hear other people's stories, we assume we're alone.

I had my daughter when I was thirty-one. I noticed a stark difference between how I was treated when I was a fully acknowledged adult who planned to continue the pregnancy versus a young college student who planned to have an abortion. All pregnant people in all situations should be supported and respected, but that's not the case, because abortion stigma is tied in messy knots with racism, classism, and misogyny.

Shame shouldn't be the price we have to pay for having abortions.

No, you're not going to hell

Religious people have abortions! In fact, *most* people who have abortions are people of faith. It's undeniable that the anti-abortion movement is deeply entwined with Christianity, but being anti-abortion wasn't even a *thing* for most Christians until the mid-twentieth century. And despite what you might think, Christians (including Catholics) have abortions at the same rate as everyone else.

Religion and abortion are not inherently at odds—faith communities of all kinds can and do affirm abortion. Organizations and coalitions including Ad'iyah Collective, Catholics for Choice, Jewish Abortion Access Coalition, Just Texas, Reproductive Agency Honoring Impacted Muslims (RAHIM), and Religious Community for Reproductive Choice organize, offer trainings, and provide direct support. They know that you are not any less deserving of support from your community because you need abortion care.

Faith Aloud operates a Spiritual Care Line (see Resources), offering support without judgment from spiritual care counselors who represent diverse faith backgrounds and are trained to support people across religious denominations.

If you are a person of faith and want to support other people of faith who have abortions, the Religious Community for Reproductive Choice offers tools and guidance for faith leaders, activists, clergy, and others in helping professions who provide spiritual and emotional support.

Digital Safety

Though abortion is medically very safe, many people are at risk of being criminalized for having one depending on their circumstances. Sometimes prosecutors criminalize people under laws specifically designed to target people who have abortions, and sometimes they twist unrelated laws for this purpose. Individual risk levels vary based on where you live, who you live with, and what information you share with others. In some cases, it's not safe for the people around you to find out anything about your pregnancies or abortions. The majority of people who are criminalized for having abortions are reported either by someone they know or by a healthcare worker. Here are some general tools to help keep yourself safe:

Use an encrypted messaging app, like Signal.

Don't use social media, email, or text messages to share information about your abortion with anyone.

Make sure to clear your website browser history, or better yet, use a browser that doesn't save or track it (like DuckDuckGo or Firefox Focus).

Delete your call history or use Google Voice to make calls.

//////////////////////

Use a period tracking app that doesn't share your information, like Euki.

//////////////////////

Turn off location services on your phone when you're at the clinic—anti-abortion organizations sometimes use geotagging to target people with ads full of misinformation.

//////////////////////

Visit the Digital Defense Fund website (www.digitaldefensefund.org) for comprehensive information on digital security and reproductive decisions.

//////////////////////

Moms Have Abortions

I had an abortion when I was twenty-one, and I had my daughter when I was thirty-one. In fact, my ten-year abortionaversary (the big 1-0!) was just a couple of weeks after my daughter was born. Spending that day cuddling the (incredibly cute) result of determining my own path felt profound. We're supposed to believe that having abortions and being a parent are fundamentally incompatible. In fact, my anti-abortion ex-cheerleader cousin once (condescendingly, arrogantly) told me that my feelings about abortion would change when/if I had a kid myself.* Turns out a lot of us were told this. But if you ask us, parents who have abortions, the reality is clear—our children *strengthen* our resolve for reproductive freedom.

**Note: My feelings didn't change.*

And get this, cuz: Most people who have abortions are already parenting.

One more mom thing:

You didn't do anything wrong,
and I'm proud of you.

////////////////////

I'll support you no matter what.

////////////////////

It's totally okay that you feel relieved.

////////////////////

I'm so proud that you did what felt right to you.

////////////////////

Your story is safe with me.

////////////////////

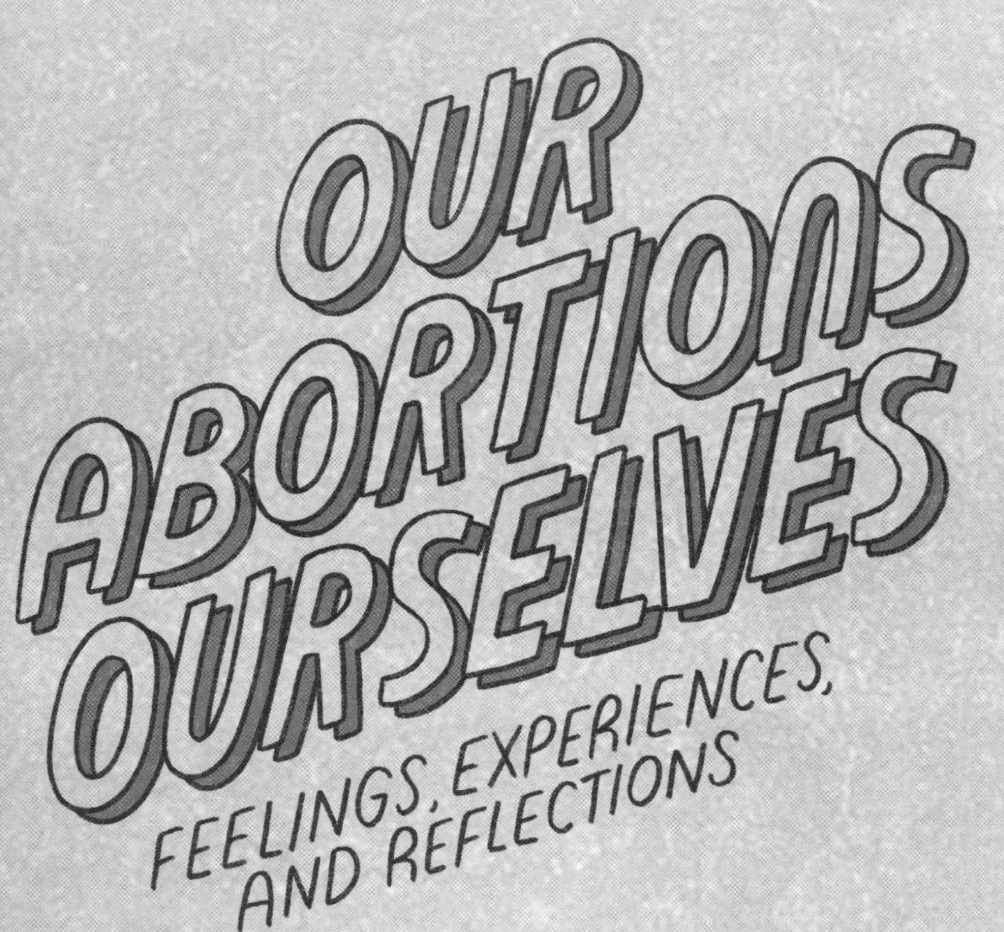
OUR
ABORTIONS
OURSELVES
FEELINGS, EXPERIENCES,
AND REFLECTIONS

"IF I HAD NOT HAD THAT ABORTION, I'M PRETTY SURE THERE WOULD HAVE BEEN NO FLEETWOOD MAC. THERE'S JUST NO WAY THAT I COULD HAVE HAD A CHILD THEN, WORKING AS HARD AS WE WORKED CONSTANTLY... I WOULD HAVE HAD TO WALK AWAY. AND I KNEW THAT THE MUSIC WE WERE GOING TO

BRING TO THE WORLD WAS GOING TO HEAL SO MANY PEOPLE'S HEARTS AND MAKE PEOPLE SO HAPPY. AND I THOUGHT: YOU KNOW WHAT? THAT'S REALLY IMPORTANT. THERE'S NOT ANOTHER BAND IN THE WORLD THAT HAS TWO LEAD WOMEN SINGERS, TWO LEAD WOMEN WRITERS. THAT WAS MY WORLD'S MISSION."

–STEVIE NICKS

Emotional Layer Cake

Your feelings about your abortions might be complex and multilayered. That's okay! All the feelings shown here (in no particular order!) are common and normal. Take a minute to reflect on what feelings come up when you reflect on your abortion. What do you remember feeling at the time? How are you feeling right now? Is there anything you hope to feel in the future?

I want to encourage you to feel your feelings to the fullest. I know it can be really hard, even scary, to let ourselves fully feel stuff, especially because sometimes it seems like we're only allowed to feel/express—or even only *capable* of feeling/expressing—one thing at a time. Anger *or* appreciation. Relief *or* grief. But our abortion experiences aren't one-dimensional, and feelings often evolve over time. There's no timeline for having feelings about our abortions. Whether your abortion was yesterday, thirty years ago, or hasn't happened yet, you and your feelings are allowed to be on your own timeline.

In my own experience, it took me a long time to unravel what my actual feelings were versus what I was told I should feel. Did I actually feel guilty? Or did I just think that I *should*? Sometimes we feel shame, not about the abortion itself, but about not living up to what we're "supposed" to feel. Social scripts about abortion are created and reinforced by things like the media, our families, and the legality of care. But you don't have to play the suggested part. I spent a lot of energy minimizing some of my feelings and inflating others based on society's expectations and the scripts I'd been given. Over time, I determined that overall, I felt really proud of myself, profoundly relieved, disappointed that my first experience with pregnancy wasn't when or what I wanted, and optimistic about my future and path.

It's Not Just Two Paths

I knew I wanted to have kids *someday*, but the moment I saw a positive test I knew that continuing my first pregnancy wasn't the right path for me. I could tell you how I was young, still in school, and in a new relationship, but none of those things mean someone cannot or should not continue their pregnancy if they want to. I just knew it wasn't *my* path, and that was that. But I've still wandered down it in my mind. I've calculated dates for birthday parties and imagined being a hot young grandma. Before I had the abortion, when I was still pregnant, I spent a lot of time mourning possibilities. I found it really uncomfortable saying no to a path in such a definitive way.

So I want you to know that it's okay to reflect on what that path might have been like and to hold space for the what-if. It doesn't mean you wish you had chosen it; you aren't being disloyal to the life you chose instead, and there's no one here to police your thoughts.

It can seem like there are just two paths—the one where the pregnancy continues and the one where it doesn't. And those directions are certainly very different. But there are just so, so many other choices that change the direction as well, infinitely forking paths. What if you didn't go on that Hinge date? What if you had pursued competitive ice skating?

Give yourself permission to imagine alternate realities without shaming yourself for it.

Making a Decision

The decision to have an abortion can be complex, with lots of variables. You might be thinking about your financial situation, your family structure, or your health and well-being. Maybe about timing, work, or the health of the pregnancy. Some people know instantly what they're going to do, and some people take a few days or weeks. You might want to make an appointment for an abortion the day you find out about the pregnancy (I did). You might strongly consider parenting but ultimately choose to end the pregnancy. You might be unexpectedly confronted with the decision later in pregnancy. Whenever and however you decide, it's okay.

If you've had a conversation about abortion with someone who hasn't had an abortion, you might have heard them say something like, "I don't care if other people have abortions, but I could never have one myself." You might have even said it yourself (before I had an abortion, I did!). So let's break it down: By saying this when we haven't had abortions, we're drawing an unnecessary and stigmatizing difference between *us*—the kind of people who would not have an abortion—and *them*—the kind of people who do have abortions. This is stigmatizing, and just unnecessary. The truth is, people who say they would never have an abortion *do* have abortions! You never know what you'll do until you're in that situation.

Some people want to talk the decision through with their loved ones or a therapist. Others might not have support for those conversations in their daily life. Check out the Resources section at the back of this book for a list of judgment-free talk/text lines to help you explore all your options. If it would be helpful to read other people's abortion stories, you can visit We Testify (www.wetestify.org). And, ultimately, you don't have to consult with

PRO-CHOICE ISN'T MEANINGFUL IF THERE ISN'T ACTUALLY A CHOICE

anyone if you don't want to. The decision is yours, and yours alone, to make.

Depending on where you live, your decision might be impacted by abortion restrictions or bans. At the time of this book's publication, forty-one states have imposed some form of restriction on abortion care. If you want to have an abortion but cannot access care, abortion funds can help. Abortion funds help people pay for their abortions. They fund procedures and can also help with things like transportation. Visit AbortionFinder (www.abortionfinder.com) for information about how to find funding no matter where you live.

Whatever you decide and however you come to that decision, I'm proud of you. There's no "right" thing, there's only what's right for you.

Other People's Feelings / If You're Sure, You're Sure

Most of this book is about your feelings. But it might be helpful to have strategies for navigating other people's (sometimes big) feelings too.

First, it's super important to remember that you aren't responsible for anyone else's feelings about your abortions. (I know, *I know*. It's a hard one for me too.)

There's a whole range of reactions that might occur when you share with someone.* There could be surprise, concern, pride, or unconditional acceptance. There could be anger or sadness. Maybe even secondhand shame (again: This is *not* your problem). It can be really hard to share about our abortions. And it can feel really shitty when someone reacts differently than we need.

When I told a family member I was pregnant and planned to have an abortion, they were supportive, but they asked if I was *sure*. I was, and I resented the question. I thought, *of course I'm sure*. (Psst: If you already know what you want to do, I promise that it's not required to think long and hard about it.) Sometimes people really are projecting weird moral shit onto you, but I think that just as often, they are simply flustered and they say the wrong things. And

*Note: You do not owe anyone information about your abortion. It's entirely up to you to share as little or as much as you want to.

that's another shitty thing about abortion stigma: It makes it so most people just aren't prepped for the kind of open, loving, and unashamed conversations we deserve!

So here are some things that people you love might say to you, and some things you can say in response.

I don't think it's the right thing

Thanks, but I know what the best decision is for me.

This isn't what I expected

The whole thing has surprised me too, but I've had some time to process and I'm confident in what I've decided.

I made a different
decision in a
similar situation.

I appreciate you sharing that
with me. I'm glad to hear
you did what was right for you.
That's what I'm doing too.

Your mom told me
what's going on—how are
you doing?

Honestly, I just don't feel like
talking about it right now.
But I've been meaning to ask you—
have you watched the latest
season of Severance?

I was so excited to be a grandma.

Please keep that to yourself.

Having an abortion makes it harder to get pregnant later.

Studies have found that having abortions does not negatively impact fertility.

Abortion is wrong.

I actually have to get going because I'm meeting my friend Becca.

No one can make this decision better than you, and you don't need anyone's permission. You're allowed to trust yourself.

Q & A

So many of the things we've been told about abortions and the people who have them (us!) are just not true. So here's a little Q & A for you, with all the stigma removed.

When is it okay to have an abortion?

~~In a very specific set of circumstances.~~

When you need one, whenever that is.

What's the best reason?

~~As a last resort.~~

There's no such thing. All reasons are valid, including yours.

Who do I need permission from?

~~*Parents, doctors, the government, partners, etc.*~~

No one. The decision is yours and yours alone.

Is it safe?

~~*It's dangerous, with long-term health risks.*~~

Both procedural and medication abortions are incredibly medically safe, with major complication rates of less than 1 percent—that's less than the complication rate for wisdom teeth removal. There are no short- or long-term health consequences scientifically linked to having abortions.

How should I feel about it?

~~Remorseful, regretful, ashamed.~~

Everyone is different, and there's no right way to feel. Your feelings might be complicated, or they might be really straightforward. Any way you feel is more than okay.

Does everyone experience regret?

~~Yes.~~

Absolutely not: 95 percent of people who have abortions report five years later that it was the right decision for them.

Release Emotions into the Lake

Picture this: You're sitting on a dock at the edge of a lake. It's early morning, and the air feels crisp on your face—I might describe it as sweat-shirt weather, or socks-and-sandals weather. The golden morning light is sparkling off the water. You can faintly hear nature-y noises—maybe leaves crunching, non-annoying bird song, or water gently lapping. You're holding a warm mug, steam lazily swirling above it. You notice how the wooden dock feels below you.

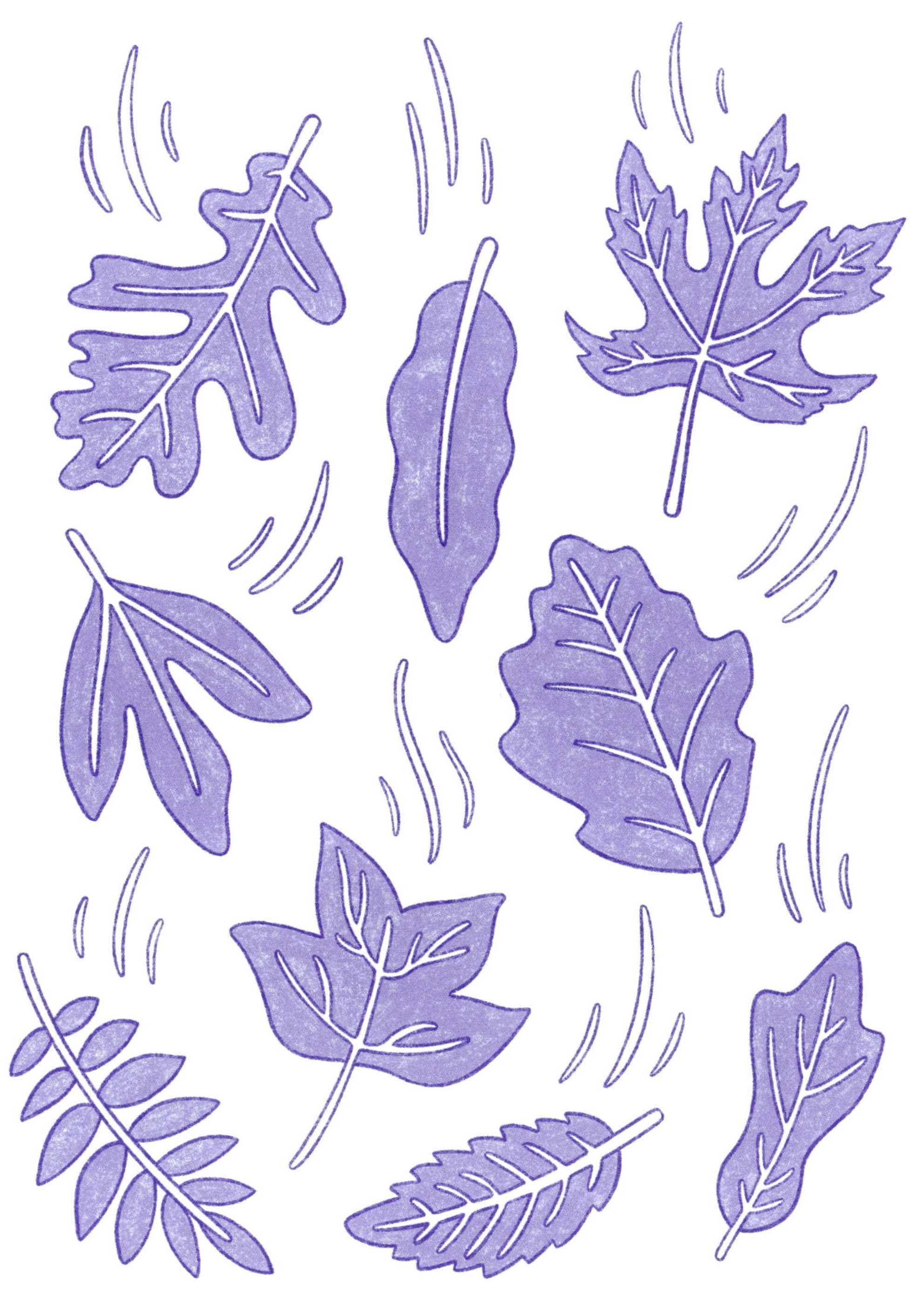

Take a big breath through your nose, exhale through your mouth. And again.

In a minute, you're going to close your eyes. But before you do, let me tell you what we're doing!

We're creating an environment to gently explore any self-critical or judgmental thoughts you might have about yourself and your abortions. You might be very aware of these thoughts, or they might be hanging out in some far corner of your brain. The goal here isn't to think *very hard* about things. The goal is to meet whatever thoughts come and then let them float on by. To invite them in, rather than shove them down. To watch them move on, rather than internalize them as fact. You're here to observe, not to *do*.

Maybe the thoughts that come up sound something like this:

I should've known better.

It's all my fault.

I shouldn't be having such a hard time with this.

I ruined everything.

I feel guilty for not feeling guilty.

I should've realized earlier.

I did something wrong.

I'm weak for feeling like this.

This makes me a bad person.

I'll never be able to enjoy having kids now.

I'm being selfish.

Maybe they're completely different. But when you notice one coming up, picture it as a leaf, gently floating down from a tree above. Maybe it lands on your shoulder. Maybe it lands on the dock next to your right hand. Pick up the leaf and hold it by the stem. Notice the shape, colors, and veins.

Spend a few moments just existing in the same space as the thought. Notice any sensations that show up in your body, like a tightening in your shoulders or a tingling in your cheeks. When you're ready, visualize the leaf drifting from your outstretched hand down onto the water's surface. Watch the thought drift farther and farther out, until you lose track of it and find yourself gazing at the flickering horizon instead.

Stay here for as long as it feels right. Take another big breath in, big breath out. Open your eyes.

Anger Meditation

The social script is that we're not supposed to be angry about what we're forced to go through when we make our reproductive choices (or anything, actually). We're supposed to be grateful for the bare minimum—for crumbs. So it's really important to me to acknowledge how fucked up it is that we have to deal with any of this at all. It's infuriating! I want to make space for that anger and give it somewhere to go.

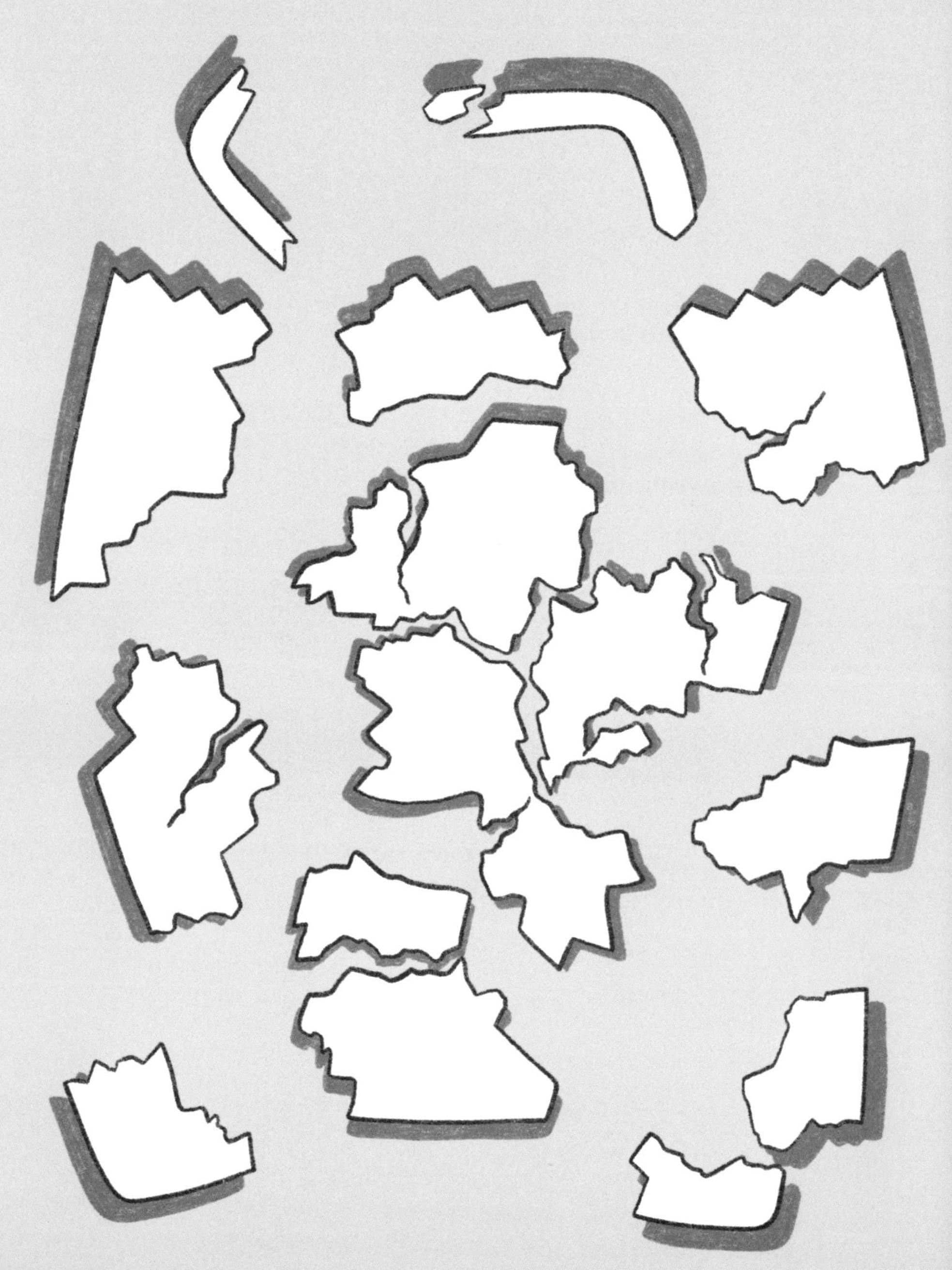

Identify somewhere you feel comfortable and won't worry about being disturbed—probably somewhere you can shut the door. Now, grab something you can rip into pieces.

Maybe that random magazine that showed up at your house addressed to someone else, your child's discarded construction paper, or a giant paper grocery bag (that's what I tested this with). Settle in, then invite the anger to join you. Personally, I like to take the pressure off by picturing my anger as a striped and shaggy-furred *Monsters, Inc.*-esque character shuffling over and plopping down beside me. Mad, but approachable.

Let yourself make space for how much easier it could have been—how much easier it *should* have been. Maybe you can identify other layers, like resentment or betrayal. Can you feel something welling up in your chest? Okay, let's get started.

I don't care what the pieces look like! You might be in the mood to make a million small pieces, or you might feel most satisfied with longer rips straight down the page. Experiment. And while you're ripping, I want you to say some things out loud, preferably loudly. The things you'll say are unique to you and your experiences, but here are some ideas to get you started:

I fucking hate Brett Kavanaugh.

//////////////////////

I can't believe I have to deal with this garbage.

//////////////////////

It's ridiculous that someone else thinks they know what I should do—literally how dare they?

//////////////////////

It's all so hypocritical!

//////////////////////

I should never have had to travel to find abortion care.

//////////////////////

I deserved so much better from [person/group/organization/movement/anything].

//////////////////////

It's total bullshit that I'm supposed to feel ashamed about the best decision I've ever made for myself.

//////////////////////

Visualize the anger flowing from your fingers onto the paper. Visualize it dispersing with each shred. When you feel things are sufficiently shredded, take a couple of big breaths. Let out a long sigh. Watch the anger monster exit the room.

Your anger is so valid. Thank you for expressing it.

Imagination Exercise

Imagination plays a huge role in making a better future—it's 100 percent worth taking the time to conceptualize what we want our world to look like, even if we aren't sure exactly how to get there. Dreaming isn't frivolous, it's vital! I'm so inspired by abolitionist educator and organizer Mariame Kaba's writing on this topic, and I hope you will be too:

"Hope is a discipline, and we must practice it every single day. It's about believing in your capacity to build the kind of world we want to live in, even when it feels impossible."

Now, I invite you to imagine: **What would a world without anti-abortion stigma look like?** I'll get you started. Close your eyes. Okay, now open them. Welcome to Barbieland! Just kidding, but feel free to include America Ferrera and/or Ryan Gosling in your envisioning if you see fit. Picture your own version of a dream world where anti-abortion stigma doesn't exist. To set the scene: Abortion pills are available over the counter at no cost. The information about abortion care that our kids receive at school is comprehensive, medically accurate, and affirming. All the formerly anti-abortion billboards say things like "Free abortion care 2 miles ahead" and "God loves people who have abortions—exactly as we are."

Let your mind wander through these questions. In this world . . .

What might someone say to you when you tell them you're thinking about having an abortion?

///////////////////

How are people who have abortions supported in the workplace? By medical staff? By the government?

///////////////////

How does the media talk about abortion? What about politicians?

///////////////////

What opportunities are available to connect with other people who have abortions?

///////////////////

How do we, people who have abortions, feel about our experiences?

Beautiful, huh? We deserve all of this, and more. I truly believe in our power to build it together—we already are.

"Abortion is

a blessing."

– ANNE NICOL GAYLOR

Self-Compassion Exercise

I bet you're a great friend. You know how gently you treat the people you love, how careful you are with their hearts? You validate their experiences, remind them how special, important, and valued they are, and assure them that you understand. As it turns out, it's possible to talk to yourself like that too. So let's give it a shot, through writing.

This could be in the form of a letter, an email, or a short and sweet note. You could type it on the computer or your phone, or write it out by hand on a piece of scrap paper or in your journal. There's no pressure to have this exercise look like anything in particular; just try talking to yourself about your abortion (or future abortion!) with the same gentleness and compassion that you would give your very best friend.

Here's mine:

Hey, B,

I remember how scared and alone you felt when you found out you were pregnant. You were so young, and it was a lot. I know those weeks where you were waiting for your appointment felt like all-consuming darkness (and the Iowan winter didn't help). You did such a good job determining what you wanted to do, even though you felt so ashamed. I wish I could've taken away some of that burden and reminded you that you weren't alone in your experience (you really, really weren't).

You were so afraid of what might happen if anyone found out that you didn't talk about it for five whole years. But now I see you talking about your abortion on the internet for everyone to see literally every day! Which I just have to say is one of the most radical shifts you could've made. It's clear that by helping other people feel okay about their abortions, you healed a big part of yourself. I wish you had known then what you know now—it would have made things so much easier on you.

I just want to remind you that you are a wonderful mother, and I know that having an abortion gave you the space to mother how you want to. At the time you felt like you were sending a soul back. You thought that since you didn't continue the pregnancy this time that any next times were tainted, or even ruined. After all, the messages you'd been given about motherhood didn't leave any room for elements of complexity like abortions. I know you were worried that when you got pregnant with baby Rea-Tucker you would feel disconnected or undeserving. So it's beautiful to see you embrace it, naturally and without hesitation.

I'm just so proud of how far you've come.

I felt a *big* wave of emotion after I finished writing this letter, almost like a whole-body sigh of relief. Of all the exercises in this book, I found this one the most helpful. There's simply no one who knows what you need to hear better than you. I smiled so widely imagining you writing yours!

I had no idea what I was going to write when I started; it sort of just flowed onto the page. Try not to edit yourself (a tough ask for me!)—this is only for you. Can you make room for both how you feel about things now and how you felt then? Those feelings might be the same, or they might be really different, and that's okay. Happy writing! I'm wishing you comfort and catharsis!

Shame Is a Sham

Having abortions is very common, but many of us hide our experiences because we're afraid of being judged. People who have abortions often carry a *ton* of shame, and it can be incredibly isolating. Because we don't talk about it, we feel alone in our experiences even though we're not. When I had my abortion, I'd only ever heard one other person talk about theirs. But that *definitely* doesn't mean I didn't know anyone else who'd had one!

Here's a non-comprehensive list of things you might feel shame about but absolutely don't need to:

You didn't use a birth control method.

/////////////////////

You did use a birth control method and it failed.

You weren't in a relationship.

/////////////////////

You were in a relationship.

It took you a while to make a decision.

/////////////////////

You made a decision immediately.

You were older.

//////////////////////

You were younger.

You already have kids.

//////////////////////

You don't have kids.

You didn't feel healthy enough.

//////////////////////

You did feel healthy enough.

All these examples are two sides of the same coin—there is no right answer to live up to. Given how pervasive abortion stigma is, society will try to shame you no matter the circumstances. Remember: We get to decide what's right for us, and we don't need anyone's permission or blessing.

Okay, so grab a scrap piece of paper and a pen. Without thinking too hard about it, let the shame flow, and make a list of all the reasons you've been made to feel that way. This could be in the form of bullet points, paragraphs, or just words. When you've written all you need to, read it back to yourself. Then crumple the paper as dramatically as you can and throw it in the trash.

We have abortions in all kinds of circumstances. And whatever those circumstances are for you, you deserve respect and support. You don't have to be perfect. Ahem: Perfection is a bogus concept!

Pleasure Isn't the Problem

There's a lot of slut-shaming in anti-abortion ideology. Shamers claim that you're a slut if you have sex, but you're somehow *even more* of a slut if you get pregnant. There's an underlying assumption that sex is inherently shameful and must be met with consequences. The messages we receive often go something like this:

The Lie: Consent to sex is consent to pregnancy.

You've probably heard someone say that every time you have sex, you should be ready to "accept responsibility" for it. And they don't mean responsibility in a normal way, such as your responsibility to respect your partner. They mean not having an abortion. Perhaps you've heard someone say something like "you've made your bed and now you have to lie in it." What a dark and decidedly un-fun view of sexuality.

The Lie: Consent to sex is consent to having a child.

This logic says that if a pregnancy occurs, you're simply out of luck. That there's only one path forward, and that is to give birth. They might say something like "there's always adoption," but adoption is an alternative to parenting, not to abortion.

The Lie: Consent to sex is consent to surveillance.

Sometimes it's government surveillance—for example, prosecuting people who use drugs during pregnancy. But it can also be surveillance by random people who feel they have a God-given right to an opinion about your decisions—if not a God-given right to be the decision-maker. This is how we get things like medical staff reporting people who self-manage their abortions to the police, even though they are absolutely not required to.

The Lie: Consent to sex is consent to losing your bodily autonomy.

The assumption here is that when you consent to sex you have no agency over what happens with your body after.

None of this is true, of course. **Consent to sex is consent to sex only.**

We're told that getting pregnant is our fault, and being forced to give birth is the punishment. It's not. You don't have to be ashamed about how you got pregnant, no matter what the circumstances were. You don't have to remain pregnant if you don't want to be, no matter what the circumstances are. And no one else is owed any of this information.

Sex after having an abortion can feel complicated, but it doesn't always. You are just as free to have and enjoy sex as you were before, as soon as you feel ready. If you're not ready, or if you are feeling like you never want to have sex again, that's also completely okay. For a long time after my abortion, I was in the "not ready" group. I obsessed over fictional holes in condoms and was convinced my second IUD was *also* placed incorrectly. I was terrified of being pregnant again—mostly of being dragged back to a place where I felt out of control of my body and life, back to a place of isolation. A lot of that fear was driven by societal stigma. Anti-abortion messaging can have a really shitty effect on our sex lives, making us afraid of sex and of pleasure in general.

Controlling sex and reproduction is critical to upholding power structures like white supremacy and patriarchy, so anti-abortion people hate when we're in control of our own bodies and sexualities. But the good news is, we don't have to listen to this garbage! Having sex isn't a problem that needs to be solved. Pleasure is healthy, and you deserve it.

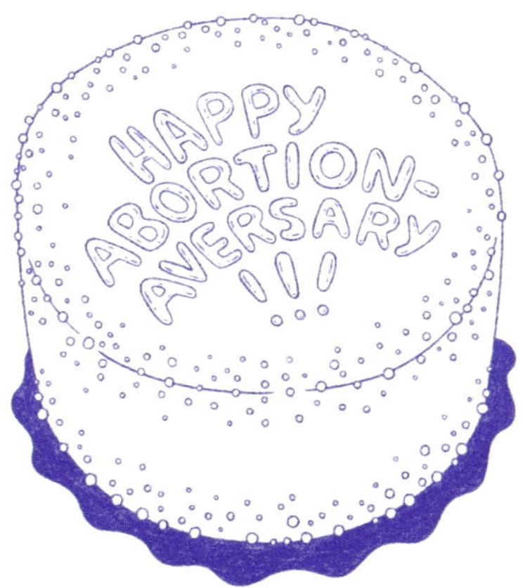

Abortion-aversaries

An abortionaversary is the anniversary of the day you had an abortion. Some people have parties, some people take time for reflection, some people feel down and need extra support, and some people don't attach any significance to the day at all. I invite you to recognize your abortionaversary in any way that feels good to you. On my own 'versary (December 7!), I focus on how proud I am of myself. And I actually choose to recognize mine on the day *after* I took the pills, in honor of when I woke up feeling like me again.

Being in a Pregnant Body / The Waiting

I want to validate how terrible being pregnant can feel when you don't want to be pregnant (and sometimes even when you do). For me, waiting to have an abortion was *much* worse than actually having the abortion. I would describe it as feeling trapped in my own body, except that my body didn't really feel like mine. If I could have crawled out of my own skin, I would have. I remember this constant, staticky, buzzing sensation in my brain.

Unfortunately, it's common to spend more time waiting than you want or expect. Sometimes people have to wait weeks—either to get an appointment or to figure out the surrounding logistics like how to pay for it and how to get there. And wait times are only getting longer as abortion is becoming increasingly banned across the United States.

Because my periods were very predictable, I realized I was pregnant quite early on. I *desperately* wanted to handle the situation ASAP, and I had assumed that I'd be able to get care that same week. To my intense disappointment, the clinic told me I'd have to wait a bit because they were fully booked. Those couple of weeks felt like months. It can be really hard to keep functioning in your daily life with a pregnancy looming over you. Working, keeping up with friends, going to class, and walking the dog can all feel impossible. It's particularly all-consuming because it's *always there*—you can't just leave your body at home when you need a break.

As with any pregnancy, there are a lot of physical symptoms you might experience while waiting, or you might

IT'S OK THAT YOU GOT PREGNANT NO MATTER THE CIRCUMSTANCES.

IT'S OK THAT YOU DECIDED NOT TO BE PREGNANT, NO MATTER THE CIRCUMSTANCES.

not experience any at all! I personally dealt with nausea, tender breasts, and headaches. I spent most of Thanksgiving Day that year trying not to vomit, and also trying not to let anyone *know* I was trying not to vomit. Trying to hide my symptoms made a hard thing even harder. If you feel comfortable letting the people around you in on what's going on with you, I say go for it. It's more than okay if you're not able to just go on with business as usual. The hormonal changes and physical symptoms in early pregnancy are the same whether you end up continuing with the pregnancy or not.

For me, the combination of physical symptoms plus feeling trapped, alone, and scared caused my mental health to take a sudden and extreme nosedive. I didn't see my friends. I ate, but don't remember eating. I went to work. I (sometimes) went to class. I became absolutely convinced that my (newish) relationship was doomed. It was really, really hard, in part because it felt like it would last forever.

So I want to remind you that the waiting is temporary—this experience will end. And I want to offer some ideas to help get you to the other side:

Move your body in literally any way.

Walk around the mall, jump up and down, stretch for five minutes.

Spend time with your friends in low-pressure ways.

See a movie, go grocery shopping together, watch TikToks next to each other. You don't have to talk about the pregnancy or the abortion, but you absolutely can if you want to.

Plan something ahead that you're excited for.

Having something fun in your calendar on the other side of your abortion can help offset the hard parts of waiting with some good anticipation. Some thoughts: an elaborate birthday party for your pet, a trip to see mountains, seeing Charli XCX live, going to an apple orchard.

Journal.

I know, I know. But it can actually be so helpful to give your thoughts and feelings a place.

A LIST OF RIGHT REASONS FOR HAVING AN ABORTION:

. . . .

. . . .

. . . .

. . . .

. . . .

. . . .

your reason
every reason

. . . .

. . . .

. . . .

. . . .

. . . .

. . . .

A LIST OF WRONG REASONS FOR HAVING AN ABORTION:

. . . .

. . . .

. . . .

. . . .

. . . .

. . . .

you're being pressured to have one even though it's not what you want for yourself

. . . .

. . . .

. . . .

. . . .

. . . .

. . . .

that's it.

What You Need

Having an abortion can be a really vulnerable experience. And it's when we're most vulnerable that we need the most support. But we don't always get it, because so often our abortions are hidden in the shadows. One of the most beautiful things about unraveling abortion shame is the opportunity to become the kind of support you needed. Every time we support someone else, we're reinforcing our own (sometimes hard-won) self-acceptance.

When I was pregnant for the first time, I desperately wanted someone to tell me that having an abortion was **not wrong**. I wanted to hear those words *specifically*. I knew it wasn't wrong, but I didn't *know*. The specific thing you needed to hear the most is different for everyone. But the sentiment is the same: I see you, and I love you. You are inherently valuable and worthy of respect.

Over time, I've collected responses from the people in my community about what they really, really needed to hear at the time. I want to share them with you here:

It's okay to believe it was the right choice.

You are a fully-fledged woman even if you never want children. Motherhood isn't everything!

You will still be a worthy mother if/when the time is right.

You are still a worthy mother now.

It's okay not to have an emotional
connection to the pregnancy.

Abortion is also a decision made with love.

Mixed feelings about an abortion are okay.
You can mourn and be glad you did it.

It doesn't matter why you had an abortion.

You're still a good person.

I love hearing how relieved you are now!

It's okay. You are okay. You are not a failure.

Your reason for this is valid.

It's okay if you don't want what is happening to your body to continue.

Whether you want support or privacy, you deserve it. This is about your needs.

I had an abortion too!

It is okay to want an abortion and still grieve what could have been.

I'm so proud of you for making the right decision for yourself.

You deserve the life you want.

You're not a killer. You're not a monster. You did what's best for you in the moment.

I'm proud of you—I know that was hard.

You can have an abortion now
and still want babies later.

There's no need to be ashamed.

Abortion can be good for you.

You are not weak and you are not selfish
for not wanting a child right now.

It's okay to be mad at how out of control
of your body you feel.

It's okay not to feel sad about your abortion.

Abortion is not selfish.

It's not your responsibility to bear this alone.

Abortion saves lives.

You don't have to feel bad
about feeling happy and relieved.

I'm proud of you. You trusted yourself to choose
what was right for you in this moment.

You're in a nuanced situation.
It's okay to feel confused and anxious.

It's all right to be really happy
you're having an abortion.

You're not a fuckup for needing an abortion.

It's always been your body.
That hasn't changed.

It's perfectly normal.
So many people have done it.
You're not alone.

Close your eyes and picture yourself (hi, younger self!) when you most needed this kind of support. It might have been when you first found out about the pregnancy, when you took the mifepristone, or days/months/years down the line. For me, picturing the shower in the bathroom where I took the misoprostol pills brings me into this headspace. And I want to tell you: I used to be really uncomfortable with revisiting these memories. You might feel the same way, so let me remind you that you are still here, safe and sound, in the present.

Take a minute to observe this other self. Are they overwhelmed? Scared? Angry? Try offering some words of support or reassurance. You are the expert on what you needed!

Compassion isn't just for other people.

Becca's Abortion Story

A big part of my abortion story is actually my pregnancy story. So: I found out I was pregnant for the first time when I was a college student, in rural Iowa, in the wintertime. My period generally arrived like clockwork, so I knew before I *knew*. I drove through the bitter cold to pick up pregnancy tests at Hy-Vee, then watched them turn positive in the shared bathroom of my group house. I googled the rate of false positives, my best friend made me frozen pizza, and I freaked out.

I knew *immediately* that I wanted to have an abortion. I was just sure. But I felt so much dread at the thought of telling my boyfriend—not because he wouldn't support me (he did!), but because we'd only been together for like six weeks tops, and I was convinced the pregnancy would ruin the relationship (it didn't!). To soften the blow, I brought over a slice of the pizza I mentioned. We hugged and agreed that everything was going to be fine.

I had no idea how to find abortion care, so I made an appointment at a random ob-gyn's office. The closest one that had an appointment available was fifty miles away. I had a transvaginal ultrasound (which I now understand I didn't have to have). They confirmed I was pregnant; I said I wouldn't be continuing the pregnancy, and they acted shocked. I didn't receive a referral to an abortion provider, and I cried in the parking lot outside of a strip mall. Back at home, I searched "how to get an abortion in Iowa." The Emma Goldman Clinic popped up, and I made an appointment for a medication abortion. This option appealed to me because I am very much a homebody and wanted to be in my own space.

While I was waiting to have my abortion, I desperately hoped for a miscarriage. My boobs were tingly and uncomfortable, and I was nauseated. I spent basically all my time depressed in a basement bedroom. Time moved so slowly. On the day of my appointment (finally!) we drove the sixty-five miles to the clinic. I thought there would be anti-abortion weirdos waiting outside, but (mercifully) no one was there. Before going in, we took $400 out of the ATM at the gas station across the street—I was on my mom's insurance, which didn't cover abortion care for dependents.

I don't remember a lot about this next part, but I do remember *The Golden Girls* was playing on the waiting room TV. I know I took mifepristone in a room with other people also taking mifepristone. I went home and took misoprostol, and at some point I started having strong cramping and bleeding. I spent several hours hanging out in the bathroom and got blood on my favorite Santa-printed pajamas. My memory kicks back in the next day, when I woke up feeling a truly exquisite sense of relief.

Your Abortion Story

One of the most cathartic things I did for myself when I started healing from the intense (and completely unnecessary) shame I had about my abortion was writing my abortion story down. It helped me to process the set of experiences and feelings that were just sort of jumbled up in my mind. It helped me to see the strength, self-love, and power in making the decision that was right for me. And it helped me to talk about my abortion (and abortions in general!) without my voice wavering. So I'd like to invite you to write yours down.

It's okay if you've never written about your abortion before. There are many of us who've never even spoken about it. The story you're writing isn't meant for anyone else! It's not a captain's log—you're not documenting for posterity, and it's not about accuracy or truthfulness. Both those things are subjective, anyway. This is just for you.

Instead of following a specific format, go with whatever makes sense for you—a list of bullet points, a journal entry, a concept map, or some kind of illustrated thing (if that's something you can do, *wow*, that's cool!). Maybe your story focuses on the physicality of your experience. Maybe it focuses on your relationships. Maybe it focuses on a specific feeling (see the emotional layer cake exercise on pages 48–50). This might flow easily for you, or it might feel pretty intense. I want you to know: There's nothing you could write here that would make me judge you. There's nothing you could write that would mean you aren't deserving of support, compassion, and respect.

That being said: If you feel comfortable sharing with people you trust and you think that would help you, I encourage you to do so.

"EVERYONE LOVES SOMEONE WHO HAD AN ABORTION."

—RENEE BRACEY SHERMAN

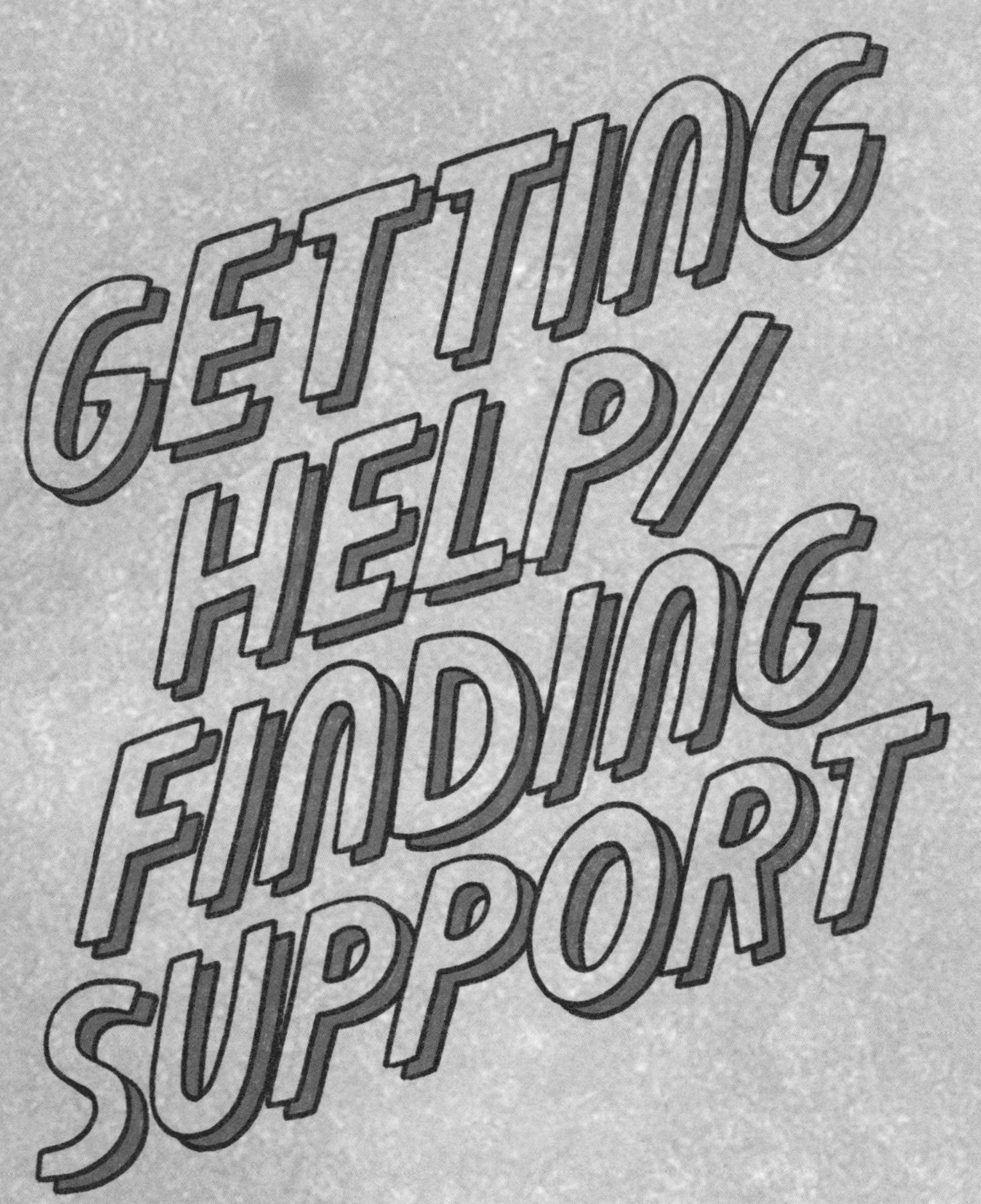
GETTING
HELP/
FINDING
SUPPORT

WE WILL ALWAYS HELP EACH OTHER ACCESS THE CARE WE NEED.

How to Ask for Help

It's common to isolate ourselves when we're going through something hard! It can be hard to acknowledge you need help, and even harder to ask for it. Maybe you don't want to feel like a burden, or maybe you're worried about being judged for needing help at all. But listen to me: You deserve just as much help as you give other people. And it's okay to be direct about what you need.

Here's some examples of things you can absolutely ask people for:

A list of shows, movies, and other distractions to binge (see page 138)

Them going to the store to grab you things

Heating pads, pain relievers, snacks, pads

A hug

Space

The juiciest gossip they can think of

Help with making sure you eat

Them going with you to appointments

Financial support

Being tucked into bed

Reassurance

A ride

Help with setting up your space
so you're comfortable

Help with making phone calls/sending emails/
responding to texts

A very long story from their childhood

That one drink from Sonic you're craving

Help with laundry and cleaning

Help with running errands

Help with childcare

Company

To make it a little easier:

Delegate. Assign someone (your partner, your best friend, your sibling) to loop in and coordinate with any other support people. Then you only have to actually *ask* one person.

Ask for contactless delivery. If you don't feel like being perceived (been there!), have your loved ones drop things on the porch for you.

Accept offers of help (try not to worry about being a burden—you're not).

Send calendar invites to helpers. Then you won't have to worry about whether they'll remember that appointment you asked them to come to.

Set up an out-of-office/unavailable autoreply for your email with a suggested person to contact for urgent requests.

I Wrote You Some Texts

When you can't find the right words to send, try some of these:

I don't really want to talk about it right now, but I'm dealing with something hard. Can you come over to watch LOVE ISLAND?

Would you mind doing a quick CVS run for me? I'm out of Tylenol and overnight pads.

Are you free Thursday morning to come with me to an appointment?

Can you pick me up from an appointment on Tuesday?

Thanks for everything today.

Remember: The people who love you want to help you. It is not an inconvenience.

How to Support Someone You Love

People often ask me how they can best support their loved ones through their abortion. You might be afraid to overstep, say the wrong thing, or that you'll do something that isn't actually helpful. From my experience talking to people who have had abortions, simply showing up goes a long way. And don't be afraid to ask them directly what they need.

If you want to help but aren't sure how, this section is for you! What would be most helpful is different for everyone, but here's a list to get you started.

Affirm their decision, whatever it is.

//////////////////////

Help them figure out the best option for care and the logistics needed to make it happen.

//////////////////////

Be a personal assistant. Help make appointments, draft emails, call people, or respond to texts.

//////////////////////

Run errands. Pick up prescriptions.

//////////////////////

Send cute pics of your pets/funny internet things/ a list of your favorite shows.

//////////////////////

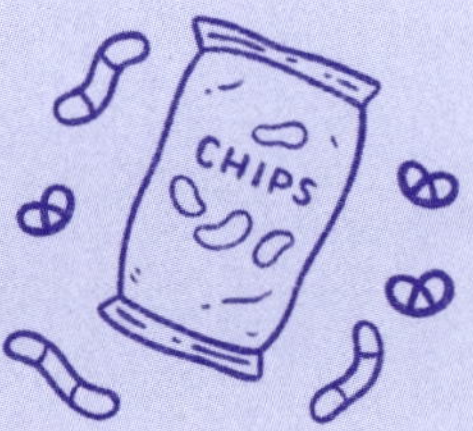

Send a food delivery gift card, drop off food on the porch, or bring snacks.

//////////////////////

Offer rides.

//////////////////////

Check in, and make it clear there are no expectations about getting a response.

//////////////////////

Provide childcare.

//////////////////////

Physical touch—hold their hand, offer a hug, rub their back.

//////////////////////

Make sure they have supplies like pads, painkillers, and heat packs.

//////////////////

Clean things or do a load of laundry.

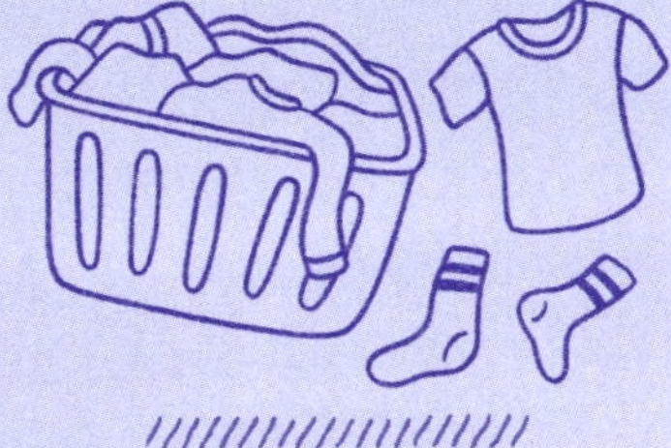

//////////////////

If you feel comfortable,
share your own abortion story.

//////////////////

Be a safe place for big and
sometimes complex feelings.

//////////////////

Reassure them that you respect
their privacy and will not share their experience
without their consent.

//////////////////

Be there. Go with them to the clinic.
Hang out on the couch all day. Just *be there*.

//////////////////

Templates /Scripts

Sometimes I struggle with sending or responding to emails, texts, and calls. And that's true in the *best* of circumstances—it gets even harder when I'm in the thick of something tough. In case you struggle with this too, let's make it a little bit easier with some templates. Feel free to adjust any one of these to make it sound like you! And yes, you can absolutely have someone else type and send these for you.

Time Away from Work

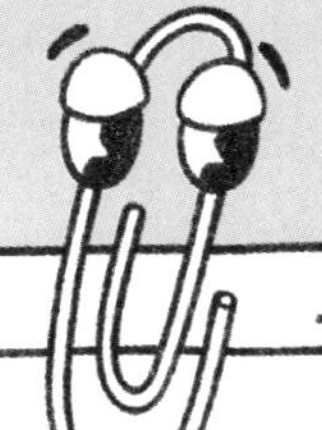

SUBJECT: Out Of Office 12/3-12/4

Hi, Anna,

I hope you're well! Reaching out to let you know that I'll be out [today/tomorrow/next Friday] on [sick leave/PTO/unpaid leave]. I won't be reachable, but I look forward to touching base when I'm back in the office.

Thanks,

Becca

SEND

Note: You don't have to tell your employer why you'll be out. If you feel like you need to give a reason, it is okay to make one up or simply say it is a personal/family situation. It is more than okay to use any kind of leave you have available.

Missing Class

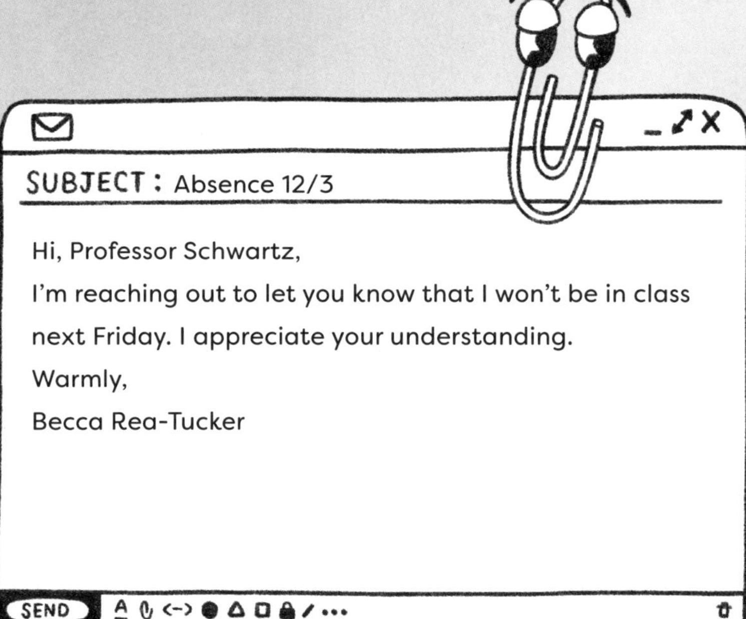

Note: You don't have to tell your professors why you'll be out.

Extensions for Assignments

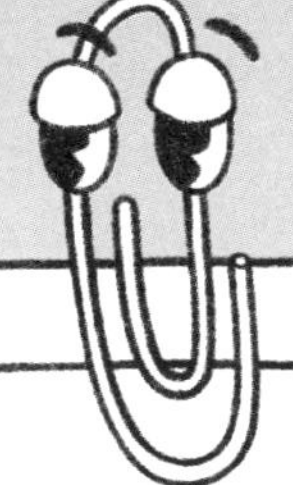

SUBJECT: Extension for REL 205 Paper Due 12/3

Hi, Professor Schwartz,

I'm currently dealing with a [personal/medical] situation and can't give this assignment my best work at this time. Is it possible to have an extension until [*date*]?

or

I'm writing to let you know that I will be using one of my two extensions listed in the syllabus on this assignment.

Warmly,

Becca Rea-Tucker

SEND

Note: I had to ask for several of these extensions while waiting to get my abortion in college. I even had to take an incomplete in a class. I felt ashamed, so I want to remind you that you don't need to. It's okay to have things going on in your life—you don't have to be perfect.

Info you might need when reaching out to abortion funds

- How many weeks pregnant you think you are/ the date your last period started
- The date and time of your appointment, and at what clinic (if you have one already)
- What kind of assistance you're looking for (ex: appointment funding, travel support, help finding a clinic)
- A callback number, and whether it's okay for them to leave a message or not

Info you might need when calling clinics

- Your name and date of birth
- Information about your insurance (if you have insurance)
- How many weeks pregnant you think you are/the date your last period started
- Whether you plan to have a medication or procedural abortion.

Also: Have them confirm that they actually provide abortion care! See page 33.

Entertainment/Distractions

I'm very much a TV person. I love lying on the couch with my giant ice water and the AC cranked up so I can wear a hoodie. I believe it's called *rotting.* And that's especially true when I'm stressed out or going through something hard. So in case you're the same way, I wanted to include a (crowd-sourced) list of comfort movies and shows for you to choose from. Note: These aren't all comforting in theme, just in result. What brings us comfort is super subjective, so choose whatever works for you!

Also: I haven't seen them all—I asked my online community to submit their faves, and these were mentioned the most.

Comfort Movies

- *10 Things I Hate About You*
- *13 Going on 30*
- *About Time*
- *A Bug's Life*
- *A Knight's Tale*
- *A Little Princess*
- *Almost Famous*
- *Amélie*
- *Aquamarine*
- *Because I Said So*
- *Beetlejuice*
- *Beginners*
- *Book Club*
- *Booksmart*
- *Bridesmaids*
- *Bridget Jones's Diary*
- *Bring It On*
- *Cadet Kelly*
- *Center Stage*
- *Chocolat*
- *Clueless*
- *Coraline*
- *Dirty Dancing*
- *Easy A*
- *Ella Enchanted*
- *Emma*
- *Ever After: A Cinderella Story*
- *Fantasia*
- *Fantastic Mr. Fox*
- *Forgetting Sarah Marshall*
- *Four Weddings and a Funeral*
- *Grease*
- *Grease 2*
- *Hocus Pocus*
- *Howl's Moving Castle*
- *How to Lose a Guy in 10 Days*
- *How to Train Your Dragon*
- *It's Complicated*
- *It Takes Two*
- *Julie & Julia*
- *Jumanji* (this one traumatized me in my childhood, but apparently lots of other people find it comforting!)
- *Jurassic Park*
- *Legally Blonde*
- *Lilo & Stitch*
- *Love Actually*
- *Love & Basketball*
- *Mamma Mia!*
- *Mary Poppins*
- *Matilda*
- *Midsommar*
- *Miss Congeniality*
- *Moonrise Kingdom*
- *Moulin Rouge!*
- *Muriel's Wedding*

- *My Best Friend's Wedding*
- *My Big Fat Greek Wedding*
- *My Cousin Vinny*
- *My Neighbor Totoro*
- *Mystic Pizza*
- *Napoleon Dynamite*
- *National Treasure*
- *Notting Hill*
- *Pitch Perfect*
- *Practical Magic*
- *Pride and Prejudice (1995)*
- *Pride & Prejudice (2005)*
- *Ratatouille*
- *Romy and Michele's High School Reunion*
- *Saved!*
- *Sense and Sensibility*
- *Sixteen Candles*
- *Sleepless in Seattle*
- *Spirited Away*
- *Stardust*
- *Step Brothers*
- *Stepmom*
- *Stick It*
- *Stranger Than Fiction*
- *Strictly Ballroom*
- *Stuck in Love*
- *Sweet Home Alabama*
- *The Birdcage*
- *The Christmas Train* (this is my contribution, it's a Hallmark-esque movie with Dermot Mulroney—I am Dermot's number one fan)
- *The Emperor's New Groove*
- *The Family Stone*
- *The Holiday*
- *The Last Unicorn*
- *The Lord of the Rings movie series*
- *The Mummy*
- *The Muppet Christmas Carol*
- *The Parent Trap*
- *The Princess Bride*
- *The Princess Diaries*
- *The Secret Garden*
- *The Sound of Music*
- *The Wedding Date*
- *The Wedding Singer*
- *Titanic*
- *To All the Boys I've Loved Before*
- *To Wong Foo, Thanks for Everything! Julie Newmar*

- *Troop Beverly Hills*
- *Twilight*
- *Under the Tuscan Sun*
- *Voyager*
- *What a Girl Wants*
- *When Harry Met Sally*
- *Whip It*
- *Willy Wonka & the Chocolate Factory (1971)*
- *Wimbledon*
- *Yours, Mine and Ours (1968)*

Comfort Shows

- *Abbott Elementary*
- *Absolutely Fabulous*
- *Anthony Bourdain: Parts Unknown*
- *Antiques Roadshow*
- *Avatar: The Last Airbender*
- *Below Deck*
- *Big Brother*
- *Bob's Burgers*
- *BoJack Horseman*
- *Bones*
- *Boy Meets World*
- *Broad City*
- *Buffy*
- *Call the Midwife*
- *Castle*
- *Charmed*
- *Cheers*
- *Crazy Ex-Girlfriend*
- *Degrassi High*
- *Derry Girls*
- *Desperate Housewives*
- *Doctor Who*
- *Downton Abbey*
- *Fleabag*
- *Frasier*
- *Freaks and Geeks*
- *Friday Night Lights*
- *Friends*
- *Full House*
- *Gilmore Girls*
- *Good Omens*
- *Good Witch*
- *Gossip Girl*
- *Grace and Frankie*
- *Grey's Anatomy*
- *Heartstopper*

- *High Maintenance*
- *Insecure*
- *Jane the Virgin*
- *Kim's Convenience*
- *Love Island*
- *Madam Secretary*
- *Modern Family*
- *Murder, She Wrote*
- *Naruto*
- *Never Have I Ever*
- *New Girl*
- *One Tree Hill*
- *Outlander*
- *Parks and Recreation*
- *Psych*
- *Real Housewives TV franchise*
- *Riverdale*
- *RuPaul's Drag Race*
- *Sabrina the Teenage Witch*
- *Schitt's Creek*
- *Sex and the City*
- *Shark Tank*
- *Shrinking*
- *Sister Wives*
- *Star Trek (any of the series)*
- *Survivor*
- *Taskmaster*
- *Ted Lasso*
- *The Bear*
- *The Crown*
- *The Golden Girls*
- *The Good Place*
- *The Great American Recipe*
- *The Great British Baking Show*
- *The Marvelous Mrs. Maisel*
- *The Mindy Project*
- *The Nanny*
- *The O.C.*
- *The Office*
- *The Sopranos*
- *The Vampire Diaries*
- *The West Wing*
- *The X-Files*
- *Twin Peaks*
- *Vanderpump Rules*
- *Veep*
- *Veronica Mars*
- *What We Do in the Shadows*

Maybe you're not so much a TV/movies person. Don't worry, I've got things for you too!

Other kinds of distractions:

- Color.
- Do a puzzle.
- Window-shop online.
- Get outside (sit on your porch, go for a walk).
- Reorganize something.
- Call a friend.
- Stretch.
- Garden.
- Garden (the other kind).
- Make Pinterest boards for every holiday.
- Plan a future vacation.
- Plan a themed party.
- Paint (art, or a room).
- Watch walking tours or *Architectural Digest* home tours on YouTube.

- Take a shower while peeling and eating some kind of citrus fruit (thank you, TikTok, for this one).
- Watch one of the San Diego Zoo live cams.
- Make a vision board.
- Rearrange furniture.
- Play the Word Master anagram game.
- Cuddle your pet.
- Get back to practicing that new language you've been meaning to learn
- Make something elaborate, like pasta or cinnamon rolls, from scratch.
- Start (or finish) a home improvement project.
- Play a game (board, card, or video).
- Craft (knit, crochet, scrapbook, make jewelry, make things out of air-dry clay, sew).

A List of Affirmations

I've had an abortion too.

//////////////////////

It's okay if parenthood isn't for you. Now, or ever.

//////////////////////

You deserve the life you want.

//////////////////////

You don't owe anyone guilt or shame.

//////////////////////

No one could make this decision
better than you.

//////////////////////

It’s okay if this was a hard decision for you.

/////////////////////

It’s okay if this wasn’t a hard decision for you.

/////////////////////

Your path is yours to determine.

/////////////////////

There is no wrong reason to have an abortion.

/////////////////////

I trust your ability to make the decision that is right for you, no matter how old you are.

/////////////////////

You are definitely not going to hell for having abortions.

/////////////////////

You don't need anyone's permission
to do what's right for you.

//////////////////////

I trust people who have abortions.

//////////////////////

You don't have to feel guilty for feeling relief.

//////////////////////

You don't have to share your story.

//////////////////////

It's okay that you got pregnant,
no matter the circumstances.

//////////////////////

It's okay that you decided not to be pregnant,
no matter the circumstances.

//////////////////////

"Abortion is about women's HOPES,

DREAMS,
POTENTIAL,
the rest
of their lives."

– DR. GEORGE TILLER

Acknowledgments

Thank you to everyone who makes the world a better place, every single day, for people who have abortions—you're an endless source of inspiration. To my daughter—I wrote this book while you napped. Thank you for being a good sleeper and the very best part of my life; I love you so much. To my sister, Isabel, the smartest person I know. To Aarti, Sam, Adriana, Alicia, and Anna—thank you for your constant support and friendship. To my mom, Melinda, and my grandmas—thanks for showing me how to blaze trails that don't exist yet. To Rhys—our life together is so beautiful. To my neighbors, for caring for us so well. To my agent, Nicole Cunningham—there's no way this book would exist without you. I'm so grateful for your unwavering support and the thoughtful ways you shaped and nurtured this idea. To my editor, Shannon Kelly—thank you for going to bat for this book. You saw my vision and brought it to life. To Dr. Ghazaleh Moayedi, thank you for reviewing my Abortion 101 section (and for everything else you do). To the books that came before this one, like 1997's *The Abortion Resource Handbook* by K. Kaufmann. To the Emma Goldman Clinic, for my abortion.

And most of all: Thank you to each and every person who has shared their abortion story and heart with me. I'm immeasurably grateful for your trust.

Resources

I know this can be scary and overwhelming. But let me remind you: There are so many people ready and waiting to help you. I've put together a list for you here.

HELPLINES

- All-Options Talkline 888-493-0092
  (https://www.all-options.org/find-support/talkline/)

Peer-based counseling and support for all pregnancy experiences and decisions.

- Faith Aloud Spiritual Care Line 888-717-5010
  (https://www.faithaloud.org)

Counselors, representing diverse faith backgrounds, offer support without judgment and are trained across religious denominations.

- Miscarriage + Abortion Hotline 833-246-2632
  (https://mahotline.org)

Private, free, caring, and accurate information and support for people who are going through an abortion or miscarriage.

- National Abortion Hotline 800-772-9100 (https://prochoice.org/patients/naf-hotline/)

Abortion provider information, referrals, and limited financial assistance operated by the National Abortion Federation.

- Reprocare Healthline 833-226-7821 (https://reprocare.com)

Anonymous peer-based support, medical info, and referrals.

- Repro Legal Helpline 844-868-2812, or fill out their online form (https://www.reprolegalhelpline.org)

Free, confidential, judgment-free legal services for your reproductive life, including abortion, pregnancy loss, and birth.

You can visit my website www.thesweetfeminist.com/abortion-resources for the most up-to-date version of this list!

HOW TO FIND CARE

- I Need An A (https://www.ineedana.com)

Reliable, regularly updated, and easy to use resource for finding care and support anywhere in the U.S.

· Abortion Finder (https://www.abortionfinder.org)

Directory of trusted and verified abortion service providers and assistance resources.

· Abortion Care Network (https://abortioncarenetwork.org/)

Directory of trusted abortion care providers.

INFO ON ABORTION PILLS

· Abortion On Demand (https://abortionondemand.org)

Telehealth clinic that offers abortion care in certain states.

· Abortion On Our Own Terms (https://abortiononourownterms.org)

Resource hub for info on self-managed abortion.

· Aid Access (https://aidaccess.org)

Abortion pills through the mail to all fifty states.

· Carafem (https://carafem.org)

Telehealth clinic that offers abortion care and other reproductive/sexual health services in certain states.

· Hey Jane (https://www.heyjane.com)

Telehealth clinic that offers abortion care and other reproductive/sexual health services in certain states.

- Plan C (https://www.plancpills.org)

Up-to-date info on how people in all fifty states are accessing abortion pills.

- SASS—Self Managed Abortion; Safe and Supported (https://abortionpillinfo.org)

Resource hub for info on self-managed abortions using pills.

- Women on Web (https://www.womenonweb.org/en/)

Abortion pills through the mail to all fifty states.

LEGAL SUPPORT

- Jane's Due Process (https://janesdueprocess.org)

Help for young people in Texas with navigating parental consent laws and abortion bans to access abortion and birth control.

- Pregnancy Justice (https://www.pregnancyjusticeus.org)

Free criminal defense for pregnant people facing charges related to all pregnancy outcomes.

- Repro Legal Defense Fund (https://reprolegaldefensefund.org)

Financial support for people who are investigated, arrested, or prosecuted for self-managed abortion or for helping someone else end their pregnancy.

- Digital Defense Fund (https://digitaldefensefund.org)

Information about digital safety and security.

FINANCIAL / LOGISTICAL SUPPORT

- Your local abortion fund!

- National Network of Abortion Funds (https://abortionfunds.org)

Check out their directory of 100+ abortion funds nationwide.

PRACTICAL SUPPORT ORGANIZATIONS

- Apiary for Practical Support (https://apiaryps.org)

See the resource library to stay informed and get involved.

- Brigid Alliance (https://brigidalliance.org)

Helps people access later abortion care.

- ARC Southeast (https://arc-southeast.org)

Provides funding and logistical support to ensure people in the Southeast receive safe and compassionate reproductive care, including abortion services in Georgia, Alabama, Florida, South Carolina, Tennessee, and Mississippi.

- Midwest Access Coalition (https://www.midwestaccesscoalition.org)

Helps people traveling to, from, and within the Midwest access a safe abortion by assisting with travel coordination and costs, lodging, food, medicine, and childcare.

- Chicago Abortion Fund (https://www.chicagoabortionfund.org)

Provides financial, logistical, and emotional support to people seeking abortion care in Illinois, Wisconsin, Iowa, Nebraska, and Arkansas.

- Northwest Abortion Access Fund (https://nwaafund.org)

Helps with funding, getting to and from the clinic, and a safe place to stay if you're traveling in Washington, Oregon, Idaho, or Alaska.

- Abortion Rights Fund of Western Massachusetts (https://www.arfwm.org)

Provides direct funding to folks who either reside in New England or are going to a clinic located in Connecticut, Maine, Massachusetts, New Hampshire, Rhode Island, or Vermont.

- Indigenous Women Rising (https://www.iwrising.org)

Indigenous-led, full-spectrum reproductive justice organization. Helps Indigenous families pay for and access abortion care, menstrual hygiene, and midwifery funding and support. Open to all Native and Indigenous people in the United States and Canada who have the capacity to become pregnant.

- Later Abortion Initiative (https://laterabortion.org)

Organization dedicated to destigmatizing and increasing access to later abortion.

EMOTIONAL SUPPORT

- 2+ Abortions Worldwide (2PlusAbortions.com)

A collection of stories from and resources for people who have more than one abortion.

- Dopo Abortion Support (https://www.wearedopo.com)

Offers a directory to find an abortion doula, someone who supports you before, during, and/or after an abortion.

- Ad'iyah Collective (https://www.adiyah.community)

Abortion, miscarriage, and stillbirth support for Muslims, by Muslims.

- Catholics for Choice
(https://www.catholicsforchoice.org)

Affirming testimonies.

- Shout Your Abortion (https://shoutyourabortion.com)

An organization that works to normalize abortion and elevate safe paths to access, regardless of legality.

- We Testify (https://wetestify.org)

An organization dedicated to the leadership and representation of people who have abortions, increasing the spectrum of abortion storytellers in the public sphere, and shifting the way the media understands the context and complexity of accessing abortion care.

WHERE TO DONATE

Your local abortion fund or practical support fund, where your money directly helps people who need abortions.

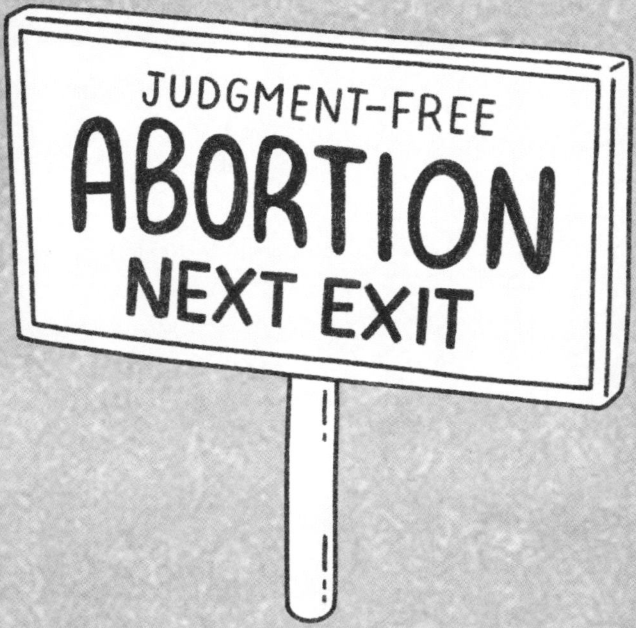

JUDGMENT-FREE
ABORTION
NEXT EXIT

Selected Bibliography

HISTORICAL TIMELINE SOURCES

Bracey Sherman, Renee, and Regina Mahone. *Liberating Abortion: Claiming Our History, Sharing Our Stories, and Building the Reproductive Future We Deserve.* Amistad, 2024.

Guttmacher Institute. "Induced Abortion in the United States." September 2019. https://www.guttmacher.org/fact sheet/induced-abortion-united-states.

Guttmacher Institute. *The Hyde Amendment: A Discriminatory Ban on Abortion Coverage.* Last modified August 2021. https://www.guttmacher.org/fact-sheet/hyde-amendment.

Kaiser Family Foundation. "The Mexico City Policy: An Explainer." Last modified August 2019. https://www.kff.org/global-health-policy/issue-brief/the-mexico-city-policy-an-explainer/.

Liu, Edward C., and Wen W. Shen. *The Hyde Amendment: An Overview.* IF12167. Congressional Research Service, 2022. https://crsreports.congress.gov/product/details?prodcode=IF12167.

Mohr, James C. *Abortion in America: The Origins and Evolution of National Policy, 1800–1900*. Oxford University Press, 1978.

Reagan, Leslie J. *When Abortion Was a Crime: Women, Medicine, and Law in the United States, 1867–1973.* University of California Press, 1997.

Texas Senate Bill 8 (2021).

U.S. Freedom of Access to Clinic Entrances Act (FACE Act). 18 USC 248. https://www.justice.gov/crt/protecting-patients-and-health-care-providers.

U.S. Food and Drug Administration. "Approval Letter for Mifeprex (Mifepristone)." September 28, 2000. https://www.accessdata.fda.gov/drugsatfda_docs/appletter/2000/20687appltr.htm.

U.S. Food and Drug Administration. "Misoprostol (marketed as Cytotec) Information." Last modified December 2018. https://www.fda.gov/drugs/postmarket-drug-safety-information-patients-and-providers/misoprostol-marketed-cytotec-information.

U.S. Supreme Court. Bellotti v. Baird. 443 U.S. 622 (1979).

U.S. Supreme Court. Dobbs v. Jackson Women's Health Organization. 597 (2022).

U.S. Supreme Court. Harris v. McRae. 448 U.S. 297 (1980).

U.S. Supreme Court. Planned Parenthood v. Casey. 505 U.S. 833 (1992).

U.S. Supreme Court. Roe v. Wade. 410 U.S. 113 (1973).

U.S. Supreme Court. Whole Woman's Health v. Hellerstedt. 579 U.S. 582 (2016).

OTHER SOURCES

Chiu, Doris W., Emma Stoskopf-Ehrlich, and Rachel K. Jones. "As Many as 16% of People Having Abortions Do Not Identify as Heterosexual Women." Guttmacher Institute, June 2023. https://www.guttmacher.org/2023/06/many-16-people-having-abortions-do-not-identify-heterosexual-women.

Guttmacher Institute. "Abortion in the United States." Last modified June 2023. https://www.guttmacher.org/fact-sheet/induced-abortion-united-states.

Guttmacher Institute. "Monthly Abortion Provision Study." Last modified 2024. https://www.guttmacher.org/monthly-abortion-provision-study.

Guttmacher Institute. "Unintended Pregnancy and Abortion in Northern America." March 2022. https://www.guttmacher.org/fact-sheet/unintended-pregnancy-and-abortion-northern-america.

Jones, Rachel K. "An Estimate of Lifetime Incidence of Abortion in the United States Using the 2021–2022 Abortion Patient Survey." *Contraception* 135 (2024): 110445. https://www.contraceptionjournal.org/article/S0010-7824(24)00108-2/fulltext.

Jones, Rachel K. "Medicaid's Role in Alleviating Some of the Financial Burden of Abortion: Findings from the 2021–2022 Abortion Patient Survey." *Perspectives on Sexual and Reproductive Health* 56, no. 3 (2024): 244–254. https://doi.org/10.1111/psrh.12250.

Jones, Rachel K., and Amy Friedrich-Karnik. "Medication Abortion Accounted for 63% of All US Abortions in 2023—An Increase from 53% in 2020." Guttmacher Institute. March 2024. https://www.guttmacher.org/2024/03/medication-abortion-accounted-63-all-us-abortions-2023-increase-53-2020.

Maddow-Zimet, Isaac, and Chloe Gibson. "Despite Bans, Number of Abortions in the United States Increased in 2023." Guttmacher Institute, 2024. https://www.guttmacher.org/2024/03/despite-bans-number-abortions-united-states-increased-2023.

Moayedi, Ghazaleh. "What Is Actually Considered an Abortion?" Clue. Updated July 21, 2022. https://helloclue.com/articles/abortion/what-is-actually-considered-an-abortion.

Moayedi, Ghazaleh. "What to Expect in the Days After an (Induced) Abortion." Clue. Updated September 27, 2021. https://helloclue.com/articles/abortion/what-to-expect-in-the-days-after-an-induced-abortion.

National Academies of Sciences, Engineering, and Medicine; Health and Medicine Division. *The Safety and Quality of Abortion Care in the United States.* National Academies Press, 2018. https://www.ncbi.nlm.nih.gov/books/NBK507229/.

Rocca, Corinne H., Goleen Samari, Diana G. Foster, Heather Gould, and Katrina Kimport. "Emotions and Decision Rightness over Five Years Following an Abortion: An Examination of Decision Difficulty and Abortion Stigma." *Social Science & Medicine* 248 (2020): 112704. https://doi.org/10.1016/j.socscimed.2019.112704.

Upadhyay, Ushma D. "Incidence of Post-Abortion Complications and Emergency Department Visits Among 55,000 Abortions Covered by the California Medi-Cal Program." Advancing New Standards in Reproductive Health. January 2014. https://www.ansirh.org/research/publication/incidence-post-abortion-complications-and-emergency-department-visits-among.

About the Author

BECCA REA-TUCKER is a reproductive rights advocate, baker, and author whose work merges activism and dessert. She is the author of the cookbook *Baking by Feel*, and through her platform @TheSweetFeminist she shares affirmations, resources, and writing that challenges shame and anti-abortion misinformation. Her work explores stigma, self-compassion, and bodily autonomy.

Becca's viral cakes with feminist messages have sparked national conversations. Her work has been featured in the *New York Times Style Magazine*, *Cosmopolitan*, *Literary Hub*, and *Vanity Fair Italy*, among others.

She lives in Austin, Texas, with her husband, daughter, and dog.

@thesweetfeminist
thesweetfeminist.com